SURGICAL PATHOLOGY
OF THE
THYROID GLAND

By

ARTHUR E. HERTZLER, M. D.

MONOGRAPHS ON
SURGICAL PATHOLOGY

BY
ARTHUR E. HERTZLER, M. D.

Surgeon to the Agnes Hertzler Memorial Hospital, Halstead, Kansas
Professor of Surgery, University of Kansas

———

SURGICAL PATHOLOGY OF THE DISEASES OF BONES
SURGICAL PATHOLOGY OF THE SKIN, BLOODVESSELS, MUSCLES AND
  NERVES
SURGICAL PATHOLOGY OF THE GENITO-URINARY ORGANS
SURGICAL PATHOLOGY OF THE FEMALE GENERATIVE ORGANS
SURGICAL PATHOLOGY OF THE MAMMARY GLAND
SURGICAL PATHOLOGY OF THE PERITONEUM
SURGICAL PATHOLOGY OF THE GASTRO-INTESTINAL TRACT
SURGICAL PATHOLOGY OF THE THYROID GLAND

Others to Follow

SURGICAL PATHOLOGY OF THE DISEASES OF THE NECK
SURGICAL PATHOLOGY OF THE MOUTH AND JAWS

SURGICAL PATHOLOGY

OF THE

THYROID GLAND

BY

ARTHUR E. HERTZLER, M.D.

Surgeon to the Agnes Hertzler Memorial Hospital, Halstead, Kansas
Professor of Surgery, University of Kansas

238 Illustrations

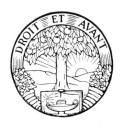

PHILADELPHIA, MONTREAL AND LONDON
J. B. LIPPINCOTT COMPANY

COPYRIGHT, 1936,
BY ARTHUR E. HERTZLER

THE LAKESIDE PRESS, R. R. DONNELLEY & SONS COMPANY, CHICAGO

PRINTED IN U. S. A.

PREFACE

THE progress of many problems in medicine may be likened to a herd of milling cattle at the approach of a storm. The animals run this way and that darting hither and yon without any purpose, for they run in circles and on the whole the milling mass does not move. Sooner or later an old maverick, with tail aloft, dashes madly from the herd in a direction he knows not of, to regions unknown, but he is going places, sometimes in the right direction.

However, this book is not as wild as it may seem. It follows generally accepted opinion, but follows them to their ultimate conclusion. If removing a part of a diseased gland is beneficial to the patient what is more logical than to assume that removing the whole will be better? To remove the whole gland is simple enough now that we have freed ourselves of the Kocher fetish of cachexia thyropraevia. It has become merely a question of technic.

I have studied my patients, removed their goiters, studied the gland in gross, and many slides stained with a great variety of dyes. I have done this many thousands of times. I have tried to write a continued story from these individual observations.

Surgeons are prone to forget that the looks of the patient, the clinical examination, the tissue in situ, the examination of the gross specimen, is as much a part of surgical pathology as the slide. The slide gives but a view which may or may not excite in the mind of the surgeon a picture of the disease process as a whole. Only a thorough study of all factors is surgical pathology. The follow up is necessary in order to determine whether or not the conclusions previously arrived at were correct.

The greatest difficulty in the study of the thyroid disease is that we have no knowledge of its normal histology and of its physiology our knowledge applies only to the earlier part of life. The physiology of the thyroid gland in the adult is in urgent need of restudy.

I have been but an amanuensis for my patients, putting down what they have told me as truthfully as possible, adding to the record such facts as the after course may reveal. That this story has led to unfamiliar scenes is obvious. The story I write is that of a family doctor who has seen many patients. Whether I am in error as surgeon or pathologist is of secondary concern. I have sought to present the premises without prejudice. The conclusions I present are unimportant. We have suffered in the past with a surplus of conclusions and a paucity of premises based on the observation of facts.

I have shifted my viewpoints often in the years but the story the patients have told are invariable. I have often thought of the words of a distinguished clinician when confronted by a wrong diagnosis: "The facts were present: our conclusions were wrong." Doubt my conclusions if you please but beware of disputing the record of my patients. My patients have been in one accord: "We will die of our goiter unless you rescue us." My "innocent" goiter patients died of failure of the heart.

As was to be expected the performance of total thyroidectomies has brought forth expressions of various kinds, notably from physiologists. The opinion generally expressed was that the whole of the gland was not removed or I do not know myxedema when I encounter it, both debatable points to be sure but a categorical disregard of the evidence here presented has its risks. I once was first aid to a venerable lady who was struck by a runaway team. She still clutched her prayer book which she was reading as she crossed the road. Her thumb nail had cut into the line "and the Lord shall lead me—." The modern version is Stop, Look and Listen.

The literary citations have been perfunctory. Since this is a record of personal experience there is little occasion to present a complete literature. I have included only a few that have been particularly useful to me.

I present the chapter on myxedema with diffidence—too little to put in, too much to leave out. That the state is one merely of diminished or absent thyroid function seems to me untenable, yet one finds cases which appear to be just that. Yet to depend on a pronouncedly minus basal rate for our diagnosis is but to read the autopsy report on our ignorance. The difficulty I have encountered in my study is that myxedema is comparatively rare. Spontaneous myxedemics with goiters, after being told by their doctors that they are suffering from a minus state, perhaps have had some improvement by the use of thyroid extract, are not crushing the box office to secure the removal of their thyroid glands.

If all the phases of a thyroid disease are considered it is possible ultimately to diagnose the condition present. Having done so I am now engaged in comparing these results with the basal rates obtained at the time of the clinical study. I hope by this means to determine something as to its value in estimating the toxicity of a given case. That its value in the clinic is grossly overestimated becomes progressively more apparent.

If this book has value it is because I have had a vast clinical experience and have been able to follow patients to a greater degree than has been possible to most investigators due to a continued residence in a small community for more than forty years.

                                                    A. E. H.

August 14, 1936

CONTENTS

ILLUSTRATIONS

Chapter II—Normal Morphology of the Thyroid Gland

xi

Chapter VII—The Cardiotoxic Goiter

Chapter VIII—Atypical Toxic Goiter

Chapter XI—Myxedema

Chapter XII—Fetal Adenomas

CHAPTER XIII—TUMORS OF THE THYROID GLAND

CHAPTER I

General Considerations

BEFORE considering the diseases of any organ it is desirable to determine as nearly as possible the function of that organ. In the case of the thyroid gland we know that it has to do with the development of the body. We know this because when it is removed from young animals they do not develop in a normal manner. We know also that when the thyroid glands are defective in infants they do not develop properly. Beyond this all is speculation. What the thyroid gland has to do, once the body is fully developed we know less than nothing. It is becoming more and more obvious that what we have assumed to be knowledge is appallingly dubitative. We do not know whether, once we have grown up, the thyroid gland be friend or enemy.

The diseases of the thyroid gland represent a wide range of disturbances illy defined from the normal and from each other. So far as the surgeon is concerned each case must be studied as an entity. He can formulate a practical conception of the disease by a study of individual cases and by constantly and repeatedly comparing the clinical and the pathologic with reference to the changed conditions brought about by any thera peutic measures that have been instituted. Any classification, therefore must of necessity be crude, elementary and, on the whole unsatisfactory, since our understanding is limited because each goiter differs from every other in some detail.

The study of any problem is facilitated by separating it as much as possible into its several parts. In harmony with this plan the disturbances caused by the diseased gland may be divided roughly into developmental, metabolic, proliferative and degenerative, though any combination of these may co-exist. The purely developmental defects, such as aberrant glands—they are not diseases—may be ignored. Metabolic changes, particularly those which take place in association with other endocrine glands, are chiefly physiologic. Our job here is to find an anatomic expression of disturbed function or functions since the surgeon's task is limited to the alteration of relationships by the process of elimination by operations.

The study of thyroid glands obtained from many sources, both from the clinic and the autopsy room, reveals certain definite changes in the structure of the acinal epithelium and often in the histochemistry of the colloid. Whether we are dealing with changes of altered physiologic

1

function, whether these changes are beginning pathologic lesion, or merely the expression of advancing years, is the first problem to be studied.

The great trouble, as above intimated, is that we do not know just what the thyroid gland is up to when we observe the various anatomic changes. That it grows us up to adult life may be accepted as established fact. As one studies all phases of its structure at all ages one suspects that, seeing its mistake after having fostered our development, it at once proceeds to get us out of the mess it got us into. Why and how we grow old has not been satisfactorily explained. My suspicion is that the thyroid gland, by throwing its gears in reverse, sees to our orderly demise, unless some intercurrent disease or mechanical contrivance anticipates its design. At least the supposedly normal gland undergoes the identical changes observed regularly in the terminal stages of the various goitrous diseases which send us on via the goiter heart.

Proliferative changes in the acinal and the extra-acinal cells furnish the earliest objects of study for the pathologist. One may accept it as fundamental that hyperfunction is always associated with evidence of increased cell activity and is expressed as hyperplasia. When these changes are present one may safely conclude that a pathologic stage has been reached. It seems plausible that the formation of new acini may be of beneficent portent, a supplement to the original acini, but the degeneration of the colloid can have no such implication. The substance that aided and abetted our development has outlived its usefulness if not its purpose. Whether this should be regarded as a normal involution or as a concomitant of disease it is impossible to say.

The clinical manifestations are so protean that, even if we knew all there is to know, they would still present many difficulties in aligning the two. Our confidence in our ability to distinguish clinically pathologic states makes us too complacent. How far a diseased condition must develop before it can be recognized as such depends largely on the experience of the observer. To say the least, disease must develop to a distinct degree before even the expert can detect a pathologic functioning of the thyroid gland.

It must be ever kept in mind that the problem is complicated because the ageing individual shows, in a broad way, certain regressive changes in the thyroid gland that are identical with those we observe in the diseased gland. Therefore, in the final stage of goitrous disease, the question is, are we observing the terminal stage of the goiter or merely the natural senile evolution of the organ which once was diseased? If this latter should be the case the only real disease of the thyroid gland would be represented by hyperplasia and the associated hyperthyroidism. We have been unconsciously assuming this and have been directing therapeutics accordingly.

Only recently have we learned that the goiter degenerates, leading to a cardiac death. Does the normal gland tend to the same end?

In any complicated problem such as this we must begin with the simpler factors and then proceed with the more obscure or more complicated. In the case of the thyroid gland epithelial hyperplasia attended by constitutional reactions, as observed in Graves' disease, represents the simplest problem.

In considering this simplest form one must include the clinical examination, taking into account all the symptoms and signs as well as the history as a necessary preliminary to the study of the gross and histologic picture: the conclusions hereby reached must be checked against the course of the disease subsequent to operations. The surgeon is fortunate in being able to study the effect on certain structural alterations by simply removing a part of the altered tissue bodily and then observing the resultant changes in what remains, also by comparing the results when the entire diseased organ is involved.

In the study of the pathology of the thyroid gland too much faith has been placed in our ability to make accurate clinical diagnoses. A clinical diagnosis is never wholly accurate. It has bewildered pathologists until some believe there is no definite relationship between symptomatology and anatomic findings. Even the most optimistic must admit that the complete life history of the disease cannot be read out of the slide—most assuredly not out of a single slide. In some cases the slide is characteristic, in others indefinite. As is generally true in pathology, the acute conditions are most easily recognized and are most easily harmonized with the clinical signs. The chronic diseases present problems arising chiefly from the fact that in their course certain changes are expressive of bygone disturbances and it is difficult to distinguish them from relevant changes associated with the disturbances at the time of examination. For instance, a Graves' disease— the most typical of thyroid diseases— in its later stages may be confused with degenerative stages which clinically may find expression in the signs of myxedema.

The first difficulty we encounter in the study of the thyroid gland diseases is the problem of morphology. We do not know the normal histology of the gland, particularly its histology in the various ages. We assume that the thyroid gland is normal if we discover no signs of disease during the clinical examination. Such an error is especially likely if we examine glands of patients who died of other diseases. If the patient was not thyrotoxic before or during his fatal illness we assume that the thyroid gland was normal. It has already been mentioned that much confusion has resulted from the pathologist accepting the diagnosis of the surgeon. If he reports toxicity, for instance, the pathologist who finds nothing to account for it, despairs of the whole problem. The surgeon may have mistaken symptoms of some other disease for the manifestations of a thyrotoxic state. It is necessary in such cases to reconsider the clinical findings anew. By following the course after operation, light may be thrown on the clinical diagnosis. It may be discovered that what appeared to be signs of thyroid toxicity were manifestations of a nervous disorder wholly unrelated to thyroid disease. Any study less comprehensive than this must leave us in confusion. It is often necessary to follow the patient for many years in order to determine the cause of the symptoms. In the fullness of the years it usually develops that the patient was right and our interpretation of the slide was wrong because the decision was premature. The pathologist who fails to find evidence of the disease designated by the surgeon should declare the clinical diagnosis to be defective instead of assuming some infraction of pathologic laws. Such a bold stand on the part of pathologist does much to instill caution into the surgeon's mind.

As in any other very chronic disease the anatomic changes characteristic of certain stages of dysfunction may be so obscure that it becomes difficult to judge the accuracy of the clinical diagnosis. Then it is the pathologist's turn to become cautious. Thus a Graves' disease established on an old colloid goiter may show in some areas changes characteristic of the acute disease whereas the greater part of the gland may present only the old chronic disorder. If there is disharmony between the clinical diagnosis and the pathologic finding further study in both directions is needed.

Generally speaking we have been hitherto concerned chiefly with the toxic states of the thyroid gland and have generally ignored the effect of the disease on the constitution, especially on the heart. Formerly the surgeon confronted by a toxic patient removed a part of the thyroid gland, the amount removed being regulated quite as much by his technical skill as by the probable needs of the patient. If the toxicity lessened he believed that he had achieved the desired result.

Having thus operated on patients in the past we are finding out to our chagrin that those on whom we operated five, ten or twenty years ago, though relieved of their toxicity are now coming to us with goiter hearts. We removed enough of the gland to control the thyrotoxic state but left enough to produce a toxic heart in later life. We only subdue the major symptoms without eliminating the menace to the patients.

Consequently it is necessary to study carefully the tissue removed for it tells us the nature of what was left behind for obviously generally speaking it is the same as the part that was removed. What effect will the remaining part ultimately have on the constitution of the patient? That question

The picture is further confused by the careless manner in which we use the term "toxic." When properly used the term must denote a physical condition associated with an increased metabolism. Nervousness, indeterminate loss of weight, rapid heart and emotional states are not necessarily indicative of primary thyroid disturbances though they are our most reliable evidence. We must consider the possibility that any or all of these signs may be due to other causes.

The problem has been complicated by indifferent anatomic examination. In many instances the gland shows one histologic picture in one area and quite a different one in another. In practice, therefore, if the part of the gland from which the slide was obtained is not in harmony with the clinical picture, examination of other areas is imperative. Obviously the pathologist has no license to say what the gland shows, but merely what the slide he examined showed. A knowledge of the characteristic picture of a certain clinical state will often induce the pathologist to continue his examinations.

Conversely, if a really thorough examination of the gland in the laboratory fails to confirm the clinical opinion, it is the clinician's turn to reexamine his premises. In the mean time events may have occurred which bring enlightenment regarding the patient's complaints.

When both methods fail of coindication we are obliged to conclude that our fundamental knowledge is somehow defective. Such cases should be set aside as unfinished business. Their accumulation may, by showing various slightly different angles, enable us to cope with some of them.

Having stressed the impossibility of classifying goiters we now proceed to do so. It is the purpose here to present the generally accepted classification in order that the beginner may have a general outline of the various stages which it will be the purpose of the succeeding chapters to elucidate. We must think of the classification as comparable to the "weeks" in the course of typhoid fever or the stages of red and gray hepatization in pneumonia; not representative of separate diseases, not even definite statements of the stage, yet in a broad way useful in the clinic.

We may begin with the classification accepted by the American Society for the Study of Goiter:

    I. Nontoxic Diffuse

    II. Nontoxic Nodular

    III. Toxic Nodular

    IV. Toxic Diffuse

The first three of these represent a degenerative state. As evidence of toxicity develops we must recognize that it is a toxicity of degeneration in which the entire gland is taking part. These changes are associated with certain variations and substages, particularly terminal, which may be called degenerative or cardiotoxic. The cardiotoxic really should form the fourth member of this group because it is the natural sequence of the other three stages. The diffuse toxic, synonymous with Graves' disease on the other hand, represents a wholly different pathologic process. It is characterized by hyperplasia and the toxicity is due to this evident excess gland activity. We have therefore two great groups. The one made up of the first three represents a toxicity of degeneration, while the fourth member, the toxic diffuse, intended to be synonymous with Graves' disease, is a toxicity of proliferation.

Tumors of the thyroid gland, including the fetal adenomas, occupy a separate place in pathology since they are not goiters in the ordinary sense, though they may be implanted on a goiter, and may produce a big neck.

It is the purpose to discuss here these several groups in the attempt merely to bridge the gap between the general principle just set forth and a more detailed consideration of them in the chapters to follow. Lest I forget to do so, I may say at the outset the idea is to emphasize the fact that goiter, whatever the type in the beginning, is a continuous process ending in a cardiotoxic state.

The Nontoxic Diffuse. This type of goiter obviously has to do with a thyroid gland that is equally enlarged in all its parts and one that causes no notable constitutional disturbance. It means that to palpation the goiter seems to be uniformly enlarged. It should imply that the enlargement of the thyroid is due to distention of individual acini, not to formation of new acini or other cellular changes. This is the only goiter that can enlarge uniformly. Because there is no cellular proliferation this type of goiter is capable of anatomic recovery. Only when considered in this restricted sense is the separation of a definite group justified.

It is distinctly the goiter of adolescence; for only in persons not fully developed do we find goiters which supply these fundamental requirements, since once hyperplasia begins the goiter ceases to be anatomically diffuse and starts to become nodular. This state, it is important to note, will not extend beyond the developmental period, for sooner or later during the approach of adult life hyperplasia will begin. In the course of time unless there is a return to normal, cellular changes do occur which may or may not cause bosselations that are perceptible to the touch. It should be noted that histologic changes occur before there is clinical evidence of bosselations. In other words, the term "uniform goiter" should signify a physiologic change only. When this stage is passed proliferation has begun; the goiter is essentially nodular regardless of whether or not it has extended to a degree sufficient to produce palpatory evidence.

The nontoxic diffuse goiters are uniformly soft and elastic and move freely under the overlying structures. If they become firm, a structural change removes them from this class even though they may remain uniform and exhibit no demonstrable clinical toxicity.

If such patients are followed throughout the years one of three things may be found to happen: the goiter may recede, never to return; it may recede for a few years and then return—usually as a bosselated goiter, especially after repeated pregnancies—and in after years become toxic; it may remain nontoxic, in so far as the metabolic changes are concerned, and pass directly to the cardiotoxic state. That is to say sooner or later they injure the heart whether they disturb the general metabolism or not.

Therefore the term is applicable in the clinic only in a general way for hyperplasia in the beginning gives no clinical evidence of its presence. Only the slide or time can tell.

The Nontoxic Nodular. In the classification these are nodular goiters because they are made up of a series of lobulations which the clinician can feel. The appearance of nodules is indubitable evidence that hyperplasia has long existed. It is therefore a purely clinical term. It has its beginning in the preceding nontoxic diffuse stages which by progressive hyperplasia ultimately produce palpable nodules. It means a nodular goiter which is not poisoning the patient, or at least not to a degree that attracts clinical attention.

The term is nondistinctive; on the one hand, because a clinically uniform goiter may be essentially lobulated on cross-section; on the other hand, because from the functional standpoint the toxicity may be present but be too slight to be measured by the usual clinical tests. The term "nontoxic" applies only to its relation to the metabolic rate. The most of them, to say the least, show some disturbance of the heart rate even when apparently clinically quiescent. It is necessary to note this fact because a bosselated goiter is cardiotoxic from the start though many years may elapse before it forces itself on our attention as definite cardiac failure. For the past failure to note this point has resulted in the neglect of these goiters until the heart has become needlessly obviously cardiotoxic.

From the pathologic point of view the bosselated type is distinctive because organic changes are expressed in terms of acinal hyperplasia. This is the important point, not the fact that they have bosselations. It is bosselated because these new acini have formed and it is these rather than the accumulation of colloid in the individual acini that are responsible for the increase in size. Therefore if we wish to distinguish between the nontoxic diffuse and the nontoxic nodular we should say the former is characterized by the absence of newly formed acini whereas the latter have newly formed acini—that is the way they become nodular. The epithelium of the newly formed acini is flat and obviously functionally not overactive.

This type may, by virtue of the newly formed acini made up of more active cells, become toxic in a metabolic sense and form a bridge to the changes which characterize the diffuse toxic, that is to say, Graves' disease. In fact in rare cases a hyperplastic toxic goiter may be implanted on a previously nodular goiter.

The nodular nontoxic goiter in the clinic, and more especially in the operating room, is composed of a number of more or less easily recognized nodules. This is the only anatomic excuse there is for assigning these to a separate class, for it is nodular or not depending on what the surgeon thinks it is. Nevertheless it is a very useful clinical classification since it brings home to the surgeon who is unfamiliar with the early anatomic changes, the fact that the stage is past where resumption of normalcy might occur, and that only operative removal can save the patient from a toxic stage and ultimately a goiter heart.

The Toxic Nodular Goiter. In the clinical sense as above noted, this type is the descendant of the foregoing group. What makes it toxic? When surgeons think of toxicity it is in terms of a boost in the basal metabolic rate. Many withhold their fire when such fails to appear. Increase of basal rate is an expression of increased metabolism which is in turn the result of acinal hyperplasia.

Usually when a nodular nontoxic goiter becomes toxic there is no epithelial hyperplasia and the pathologist despairs. The fact is, in the majority of cases there is no hyperplasia. It is a toxicity of degeneration. If one studies these goiters carefully the colloid is found to have become basophilic, the cells flat, the nuclei stain variously and in many the connective tissue has undergone change. The patient is sick and there is no evidence of cellular hyperplasia, but there is abundant evidence of degeneration. One is compelled to say that it is a toxicity of degeneration.

There are cases in which the increasing toxicity is a sign of augmentation of the hyperplastic process. These show evidence of toxicity in the laboratory by the presence of increased hyperplasia and a palely staining acidophilic colloid. This represents a bridge between the colloid and the hyperplastic toxicity. Sometimes the pathologic study is confused by the fact that only a part may be hyperplastic and a cursory examination fails to locate it.

The fundamental question to the surgeon, therefore, is just how toxic must the patient be before the goiter should be classed as toxic. The excessive thyroid secretion manifests itself by increased pulse rate and nervousness and loss of weight. Yet the patient may be toxic without these signs being manifest. The toxicity of degeneration may find its expression in general disturbances, fatigability and cardiac manifestations. These prove as perplexing to evaluate in the clinic as in the laboratory. It is difficult to express these gradual changes in clinical terms. This is the reason some pathologists have abandoned all attempts to harmonize the pathology with the clinical findings. If he will calm himself he will immediately discover that he has been trying to paint a pathologic picture from the design of the clinician and not from the physical condition of the patient. Just here is the crux of the whole thing. The problem cannot be treated as abstract. Each patient is a concrete problem and must be studied, not only continuously, but simultaneously in the clinic and the laboratory. It is distinctly a one man's job, or at least a close association between the surgeon and pathologist and is effective when each fully understands the problems of the other. It cannot be accomplished so long as the surgeon hands the pathologist the tissue on the end of a stick, as is generally done.

There are yet other difficulties besides those of correctly correlating the clinical and the anatomic. The functional changes, more labile than the anatomic, may intervene to add complications. If the goiter be functionally active the slide may show too little, if functionally low, too much. One could observe this in the old days of pole ligation; a removal of a wedge of tissue showed a certain pathologic picture. After some weeks or months the patient displayed great clinical improvement, and a lobectomy was done but the slide of the gland removed then looked just like the section obtained from the tissue removed at the time of pole ligation. One can see much the same thing in two-stage lobectomies. One lobe removed shows a certain picture; great clinical improvement follows. When the second lobe is removed there is the same picture. This proves merely that there is a functional complication we have not found in the slide. I believe it is to be found in the histochemistry of the colloid.

The picture may be complicated when the sluggishly toxic goiter suddenly becomes violently toxic, accompanied with marked loss of weight, tremor; even eye signs may occur. These have been called Basedowified colloid goiters. In other words a new type of toxic goiter. These moderately degenerated toxic nodular goiters which have already reached a state of cardiac involvement when complicated epithelial hyperplasia may suddenly degenerate and produce high fever, delirium; exfoliated endothelium, death. The degenerative toxic changes when complicated with epithelial degeneration produce the most violent terminal states.

Diffuse Toxic Goiters. This term is used as a synonym for Graves' disease and exophthalmic goiter. They are hyperplastic and the toxicity is due to hypersecretion. They are not preceded by a colloid goiter hence are not complicated by a pre-existing toxicity of degeneration.

This type as the name implies is uniformly enlarged and is toxic. It is uniform, at least as uniform as a normal thyroid because it begins in early life when all goiters, generally speaking, are uniform. It is uniformly enlarged because the disease develops principally from hyperplasia of the epithelium in the original acini and does not await more leisurely process of accumulation of colloid in the acini.

Whether or not a nontoxic goiter always precedes the toxic state is not known. Certainly they may quickly develop in a thyroid gland not previously recognized as enlarged. "Primary toxic," therefore, would appear to be an enlightening synonym in many cases. Generally, especially in children, it is obvious that there was a preceding colloid goiter and that for unknown causes, hyperplasia suddenly developed.

This group is as distinctive in the clinic as in the laboratory. It is characterized by vascular changes, tremor, rapid and extreme loss in weight, hard, uniform gland. In some there are eye signs. These are the true Basedows. The tendency is to run an acute course and to enter a remission after a period of months or years.

Anatomically they are characterized by evident epithelial hyperplasia and a thin acidophilic colloid. Those attended by eye signs in addition to acinal hyperplasia present a definite papillation of the epithelium into the lumina of the acini.

Cardiotoxic Goiter. This group has no place in our accepted classification. It is the end stage of the preceding groups, including the acute Graves' disease. Cardiac death must be regarded as the normal result of all goiters. It does not find a place in the classification because clinical examination of the goiter fails to detect its presence. One must find the evidence in the heart. The goiter may belong to one of the several groups already discussed. Furthermore in many cases of goiter attended by cardiac degeneration the gland is small and uniform in outline. In fact the goiter may be discovered only after the development of cardiac signs send us hunting for a goiter. A goiter heart is always the result of degeneration, whether there be associated hyperplasia or not. For this reason it becomes a question whether these are not really cases of degeneration of the thyroid gland, distinctive and not necessarily a part of thyroid enlargement. It does emphasize this one outstanding fact: the most important disease of the thyroid gland is not inseparably associated with thyroid enlargement. This fact necessitates studying the thyroid from a new angle.

Tumors of the Thyroid Gland. Tumors likewise find no place in our clinical classification. And correctly, for the tumorous process is only remotely related to goiters as such. It need only be mentioned here that with the tumors belong the fetal adenomas. These are derived from misplaced bits of thyroid tissue which develop as encapsulated nodules which are wholly unaffected by the state of the remainder of the gland, whether it be normal or goitrous. The fact which concerns us here is that they are commonly confused with the bosselations of the nodular goiters.

The neoplastic diseases as such which develop in the thyroid gland generally follow the laws governing all tumors; but since their early identification is dependent on the goitrous changes, it becomes necessary to devote a special chapter to their consideration.

Literature

In the consideration of the literature of the general principles of goiter one need quote but one paper, that of Wilson (*Surg., Gynec. and Obst.*, June 1909, 9, 588–602). He writes: "In a previous communication (*Trans. Asso. Am. Phys.*, 1908, 23, 562–578) I have attempted to show that certain pathological changes in the thyroid gland have a definite relationship to the varying symptoms in Graves' disease. That such a definite relationship does exist there can be no doubt in the mind of anyone who has examined any considerable number of cases, comparing the lesions with the symptoms. . . . Finally, when glands removed in cases of previous hyperthyroidism are found to consist of acini lined with flattened or desquamating epithelium and filled with a thick gelatinous non-absorbable colloid a careful study of the symptoms of the case will show that the patient is suffering from lesions of vital organs—heart, central nervous system, etc., which were produced by a long-passed thyroid toxemia."

That paper thoroughly impressed me with the fact that in goiter, as well as all other diseases, there must be a relation between the pathology and the clinical manifestation. In fact this book is dedicated to an effort to demonstrate that relationship.

Chapter II

Normal Morphology of the Thyroid Gland

THE thyroid gland presents so much structural variation in supposedly normal persons that it is difficult to paint a picture sufficiently accurate to serve as a guide in the study of its pathology. It is at once evident that its structure varies greatly at the different ages, hence every period of life must be considered separately. Infancy, maturity and old age each presents a different picture. The thyroid gland is supposed to experience rapid changes, not only in the epithelium and colloid but even in the connective tissue in certain diseases. It must be remembered that in many cases these are merely expressions of opinion which are without a basis of demonstrable facts. However, supposing the thyroid gland to be such a labile organ and assuming that autopsy material is likely to be misleading because postmortem changes occur before the tissue can be fixed but more especially because of the effect disease may have had on the gland itself it is desirable to select for anatomic study material free from these influences. Notwithstanding these possibilities, most diseases do not seem greatly to influence the structure of the gland.

Be this as it may, in my study of histology I have used autopsy material, obtained from the bodies of those who died of some disease, only for comparison. In order to construct as accurate a concept as possible of the normal gland I have relied entirely on autopsy material obtained from those who met sudden death (from which the gland was obtained without delay), and on biopsy material secured during operations in the thyroid region for lesions not affecting the gland itself, such as operations on the larynx, sometimes in block dissections of the neck, but particularly in operations on esophageal diverticula wherein it was necessary to ligate and divide the vessels of the superior pole and in days long gone by, in doing tracheotomies in diphtheria.

Because of the alleged rapid changes in the colloid, both in health and disease, this substance has been especially studied, not only from fresh material obtained from healthy subjects but also in cases of the various diseases.

In this research a great variety of dyes and methods of preparation have been employed both in the study of the cellular elements and of the colloid. The usual laboratory stains, save in routine preliminary examinations,

14

leave much to be desired. For detailed study special dyes and methods of fixation must be employed. By these means the various structures can be made to stand out conspicuously, particularly the connective tissue and the colloid. Such a study of the normal gland is essential in order to form a basis for the study of the pathologic gland. It is necessary therefore to mention the technic employed in some cases in staining the slides from which the various figures were made. Unfortunately it is not yet possible to present these interesting studies in tinctorial chemistry on the printed page.

The basic histology is built on the thyroids of adolescents and of persons in early adult life, the ages ranging from fifteen to twenty-eight years. During that period it is safe to say that full development of the gland, as well as of the individual has been achieved. For a period of years the high point of development is maintained, but beyond a certain point certain secondary and probably degenerative changes begin to develop. There is no fixed age when these changes begin. In some cases they are observed even in the developmental period but generally they are not marked until the fourth or even the fifth decade of life.

It is necessary to have in mind the possibility of early degeneration because the great majority of goiters start soon after maturity is reached and once a goiter has begun one must be prepared to find evidence of degeneration no matter what the age of the patient or the apparent physical condition. Many pictures accepted as normal variants are no doubt those of incipient goiters or initial transitions toward degeneration which in later life will find expression in cardiac disturbances. Therefore, while it is necessary to have in mind a fixed notion of the normal gland, one must be prepared to regard any deviations from this as evidence of disease.

One's understanding of the adult gland is aided by the study of it in infancy and childhood. In fact many of the dubitative points in both histology and pathology can be clarified by keeping in mind the various developmental stages of the infantile gland. This is particularly important because many glands, like the individuals they serve, never attain an adult stage and these underdeveloped glands may be confused with those undergoing early pathologic changes.

The formulation of a mental picture of the normal gland in the later stages of midlife and old age is not so easy. First of all a senile person must be regarded as one who is senile clinically. He may be old in years without being senile physically. The thyroid registers changes in terms of actual senile changes only, regardless of the calendar age of the individual. Conversely, we know that patients with toxic goiters age rapidly. A patient aged 50 with goiter may be as senile as one of 80 years who is not afflicted with goiter. Broadly speaking I believe the structure of the thyroid gland is a more reliable guide to the actual physical age of the individual than is the date recorded in the family bible. It is a good clinical lead, when confronted by a patient who is older in appearance than the age he gives, to suspect changes in the thyroid gland whether or not it has attained sufficient size to form a clinical goiter.

Obviously then it is impossible to draw a satisfactory border-line between senile and goitrous glands because the changes run more or less parallel. We are concerned here of course only with presenting a picture of the glands of normally physically aged individuals. This is achieved by studying the thyroids of persons who were apparently in good health before the accidents which terminated their lives, and whose physical state corresponded with their given age.

In determining the actual physical age for a goiter attention must necessarily center on the study of the connective tissue and colloid as well as on the acinal epithelium, a fact too often overlooked. The changes in the colloid are even more important than is the study of the connective tissue in determining when a goiter is senile.

In order to present the histologic picture of the thyroid gland as clearly as possible it seems best to discuss aspects of the gland of the adolescent, of the adult and of the senile individual. This discussion may be preceded by a brief reference to the gross anatomy of the gland.

    I. Gross Anatomy of the Thyroid
    II. Histology of the Prenatal Child, Infant and Adolescent Thyroid Gland
    III. Histology of the Adult Thyroid Gland
    IV. Histology of the Senile Thyroid Gland

THE GROSS ANATOMY

If a sophomore were asked to describe the normal anatomy of the thyroid gland he would say that it is a bilaterally symmetrical organ formed of two lobes, one lying on either side of the trachea and united by an isthmus from the upper border of which extends a pyramidal lobe that usually reaches the height of the hyoid bone. And we would give him a ten. If a layman asks us the size of the gland it is proper to say the average weight is around 20 to 25 grams.

To the student of the gland pathology the important points are that the surface is made up of low lobulations (Fig. 1) which are noticeable when the capsule has been removed. The surface is never smooth like that of the liver and spleen. The adult gland encased in its capsule shows an undulating surface with indentations here and there which indicate

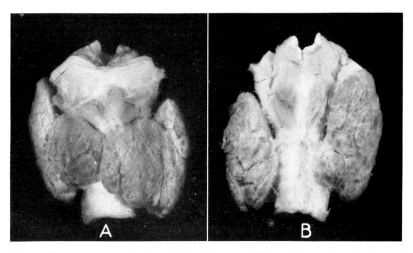

Fig. 1. Gross anatomy of a thyroid gland from a child aged three. Its relation to the larynx and trachea is shown. The capsule has been removed from the gland, showing its uneven surface and indications of lobule formation. *A*, View from in front. *B*, View from behind.

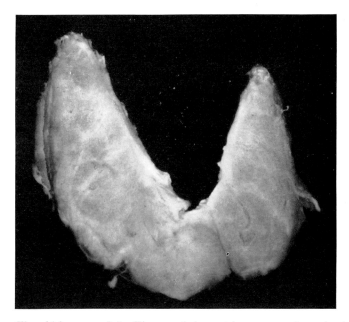

Fig. 2. Thyroid from an adult. The capsule has not been removed, partly obscuring the nodulations. Even so low bissilations are clearly in evidence though partly obscured by the capsule.

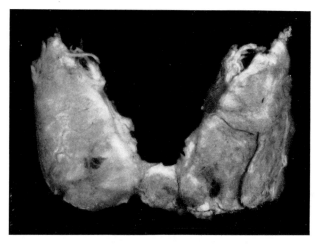

FIG. 3. Thyroid gland from an old man. It is small and fibrous terminating at the poles in sclerosed borders. It weighed 14 grams.

where connective tissue septa enter the gland (Fig. 2). The right lobe commonly extends higher in the neck than the left, as shown in both the above figures. The senile gland is usually smaller, of denser consistency, and it may present fibrosis beneath the puckered capsule (Fig. 3).

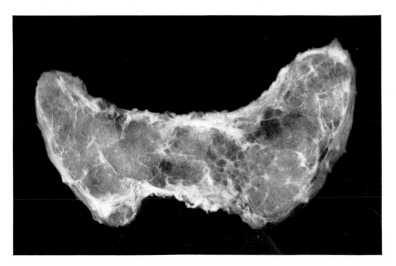

FIG. 4. Cross-section of a normal thyroid gland in a young adult. The parenchyma is divided into more or less spherical areas by the fibrous septa which go out from the capsule of the gland.

The cut surface shows the parenchyma intersected by fibrous septa which go out from the gland capsule, dividing it into fields perceptible to the naked eye (Fig. 4). These macroscopic fields are subdivided again and again, making still further subdivisions which are microscopic. An appreciation of the spheroidal fields is prerequisite to the understanding of the formation of nodules, the so-called adenomas of the goitrous glands.

As useless information it may be added that not infrequently the isthmus is a mere fibrous band and that the pyramidal lobe sometimes goes out from the midpart of the isthmus and sometimes from the lateral parts,

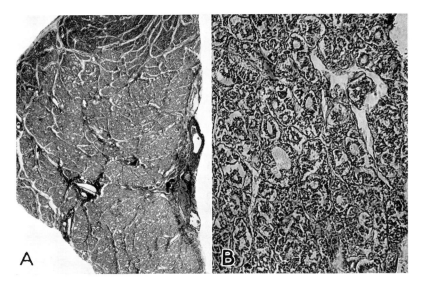

FIG. 5. Thyroid gland from a six months' fetus: *A*, shows the division of the parenchyma into lobules by the fibrous septa (×8); *B*, many of the small follicles are lined by well formed cuboid epithelium, some show scarcely any lumina at all and there are many diffuse cell masses. The colloid is finely granular. (×70).

but seldom from one of the poles. In rare instances one lobe may be entirely absent. I had one such case and have seen another.

HISTOLOGY OF THE PRENATAL AND INFANT THYROID GLAND

Embryologists know exactly how the thyroid gland is formed. This knowledge is of interest to the surgeon only in so far as it explains the location of aberrant lobes. His interest begins with the formation of acini. Since it is impossible to secure reasonably normal material until after birth, the appearance of the gland of embryos as seen in the slide must be given conservative interpretational consideration because postmortem changes occur rapidly.

The Prenatal Gland. My earliest material is that of a six months' fetus whose exit was expedited by a severe injury to the mother. The slide of this gland shows few postmortem changes. There are well formed follicles but the colloid is sparse, granular and unresponsive to any dye (Fig. 5). Even at this late date of prenatal development it is to be noted that there remain many solid columns of cells without the lumina that are found in the regular structure of the still earlier glands. I have no satisfactory

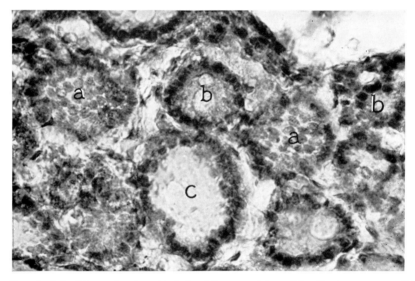

Fig. 6. Acinal formation in a fetal gland interposed by solid cell masses: *a,a,* solid columns of cells without lumina; *b,b,* beginning formation of lumina; *c,* definitely formed acinus containing stainless colloid. The cells in all of these structures stain the same.

specimens of these latter. The desquamation of epithelium shown in many published cuts of embryonal glands must be regarded as due to postmortem changes. The greatest interest in these early glands centers in the solid cell masses or very small follicles between the larger acini. The origin and meaning of these small follicles are of great interest in the interpretation of the bosselations, the adenomas, and in certain goiters of low toxicity (interstitial goiters).

It may be here stated that several theoretical explications have been evolved concerning the formation of small follicles in normal and in pathologic glands. The oldest theory is that they are formed from the same anlage that have developed into the larger colloid-containing follicles. The second theory has them developing by budding of the larger acini, two, resulting from a constriction of a larger acinus. The third and most recent view is that there are no such things as small interacinal follicles and cell masses. Proponents of this theory believe that what appear to be inter-acinal cell masses are simply the tops of acini cut across above the lumen. Ignoring the obvious physical impossibility of so many elongated processes appearing in the one area, the structure of the cell masses is sufficient refutation. The size of the cell groups made up of cells with nuclei sur-rounded by protoplasm of equal amount cannot be tangential sections

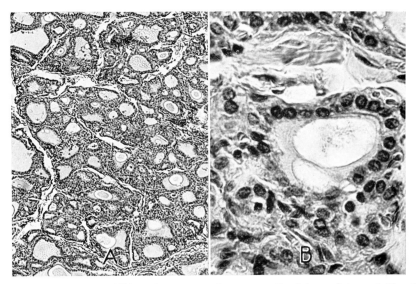

FIG. 7. Slide from a child aged two years: *A*, many small acini containing colloid and many cell masses without colloid-containing lumina; *B*, one large acinus lined with low columnar epithelium containing granular colloid. Below are cell masses without definite lumina.

(Fig. 6). In this connection it is only necessary to note that the colloid-containing follicles once were solid masses, as is shown by the fact that in early fetal life some contain colloid while others do not. Those not yet having formed lumina are made up of the same identical cells as those which contain colloid. The development of acini can well be studied in fetal adenomas since these tumors are merely encapsulated fetal rests projected into adult life for further development. This problem will be discussed further in subsequent chapters.

The Infant Gland. During the first months of the infant's life the thyroid gland differs very little from the prenatal, but there is a progressive formation of acini (Fig. 7). The acinal cells show more tinctorial differentiation between nucleus and the protoplasm. There are many acini, some without and some with demonstrable protoplasm. Also the colloid is more uniform though it does not yet attract the acid dyes.

The Thyroid Gland of Children and Adolescents. Just when childhood ends and adolescence begins it is impossible to say. It is necessary therefore to take a look at the glands representing the various ages. It can be said that there is neither uniformity as to age nor regularity as to the order of the developmental changes. The changes as age advances are, in general, attended by a lessening of the interacinal cell masses, by the increase

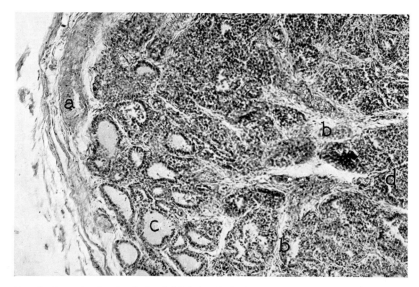

Fig. 8. Capsule of a gland of a child: it is relatively thicker than in the adult as are the septa; *a*, capsule with vein; *b,b*, connective tissue septa extending into the interior of the gland dividing it into fields; *c*, acini with lumina; *d*, cell masses without lumina.

of the size of the acini and by the more definite acidophilic staining of the colloid.

It may be said at the beginning that certain delays in development may be observed in the thyroids of children who have marked peculiarities of constitution that may be recognized in the clinic. These are not to be confused with normal glands.

In examining the various parts of the glands in very young children one is dependent largely on autopsy material and one must have in mind possible changes incident to the lethal disease, though none is evident. In older children operations on the trachea not infrequently provide biopsy material. When the automobile age is attained there is no lack of material from healthy individuals.

It is convenient to examine the various parts of the glands as entities in order to emphasize their characteristics.

The Capsule and Blood Vessels. The capsule in children is relatively thick, as compared with the adult gland, and its structure is such that it does not take the usual connective tissue dyes as does the capsule of the adult gland. The bundles of fibers are fairly heavy and stain brown with van Gieson's stain. From the capsule heavy septa extend into the gland,

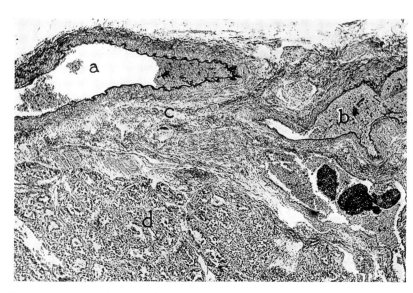

Fig. 9. Blood vessels of the thyroid in a child: *a*, artery cut obliquely showing definitely stained elastic tissue layer and thick muscle wall; *b*, vein with definite walls; *c*, connective tissue of the capsule; *d*, the acinal epithelium is desquamated due to postmortem changes.

forming more or less definite lobules (Fig. 8). From these, secondary fibers extend into the surrounding acini and form small lobules. The ultimate division where it surrounds each individual acinus is very fine. This arrangement is of course that found in the adult gland, but it is of interest to note that the arrangement is definite even in the infant gland.

The blood vessels are relatively more prominent than those in the normal adult gland (Fig. 9). This is particularly true of the veins. The interacinal vessels stand out prominently when the blood hardens *in situ* in the infant. In such specimens the blood sinuses are seen to occupy more space than the acini (Fig. 10). The relative size of the blood vessels is more impressive in such slides than in injected specimens.

The Acini. The acini furnish the most important factor in the study of the histology of the gland in early life. On the appreciation of the changes that occur during the process of reaching the adult stage depends a clear understanding of many phases of the pathology.

One's notion as to the age at which all acini are formed comparable to the adult stage depends on one's idea of the formation of acini in later life. My opinion is that some such cells lie dormant in the interacinal spaces

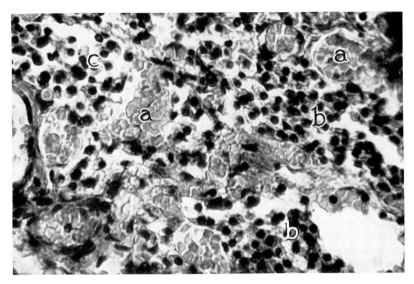

FIG. 10. Thyroid of a child, hardened in situ: *a,a*, blood channels distended with red corpuscles; *b,b*, cell columns which have not yet formed acini; *c*, scattered cells due to postmortem changes. The cells contain large deeply staining nuclei with little protoplasm.

and are capable of forming new acini at a later period of life. I also believe some of these cells may persist in a more or less infantile state and that they are capable of influencing the endocrine balance of the individual even in adult life.

If one accepts this view the stage is reached at about the seventh to the tenth year. The acini when fully developed in the child are lined by a uniform columnar epithelium or a cuboidal epithelium similar to that of a young adult (Fig. 11). A lesser epithelium is not observed before puberty. The nuclei are in midposition and for the most part stain well. The cyto-

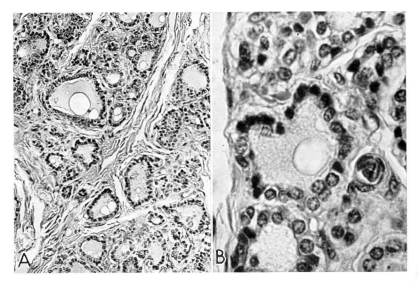

FIG. 11. Slide from the thyroid gland of a child aged seven: *A*, many acini contain colloid, some with vacuoles, and are lined with cuboid or low columnar epithelium; *B*, two well formed acini containing colloid and several groups of cells without lumina.

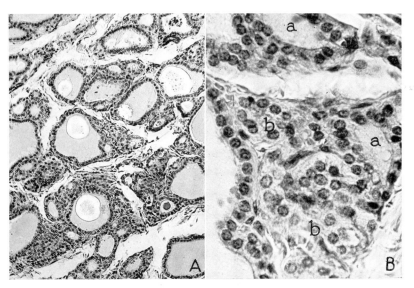

FIG. 12. Slide from a child aged six years: *A*, the acini are well formed for the most part but with islands of interacinal cells. *B*, Same, high power. The acinal cells, *a,a*, are cuboidal; *b,b*, interacinal cell nests without lumina.

plasm is uniform or granular and stains poorly (Fig. 12). The cells in the interacinal spaces stain the same as those of the acini.

The Colloid. As has been previously remarked the colloid in very early life is so thin that it is not stained at all by eosin and only faintly by Mallory's trichrome methylene blue. It does not stain normally, as compared to the adult, until the fourth or sixth year (Fig. 12). When it does stain it is uniformly acidophilic with eosin.

It is of importance to note that the gland weighs 2.5 grams at birth and 10 grams at the age of 14 years. This means that the remainder, say 15

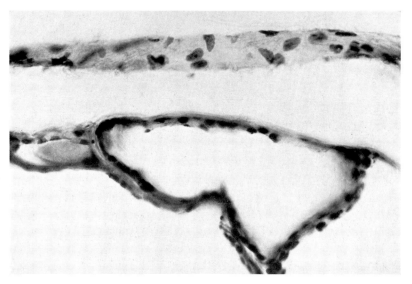

Fig. 13. Slide from a normal thyroid gland from which the capsule has been teased off. It is a sheet-like layer containing ovoid cells with small dark nuclei. Beneath are acini with flat, imperfect epithelium. The goiter was an adolescent colloid from an anemic young girl.

grams, develops after puberty to make up the 25 grams average weight at the age of 28 years. This is of interest because the thymus has long since become regressive. Broadly speaking, the opinion may be ventured that the thyroid assumes dominance after the regression of the thymus, in the development in the latter part of adolescence. The slow development of the thyroid gland is of interest in determining how long the gland is vitally important in the development of the individual.

THE ADULT GLAND

As the age when the adult gland is typical, 28 years may be taken, though there is no notable variation for some years prior or subsequent thereto. This age is free from the associated endocrine changes incident to puberty and there are few changes inseparable from diseased or senile states. During this period, however, one does find glands which show structures generally found only in the child, notably the interstitial cells, and particularly, colloid changes common to advanced years.

Here, as in the case of the adolescent thyroid glands, the capsule, the acini and the colloid may be discussed as entities.

The Capsule. The gland has a thin capsule of white connective tissue when seen in the gross. The slide shows this to be made up of flat and

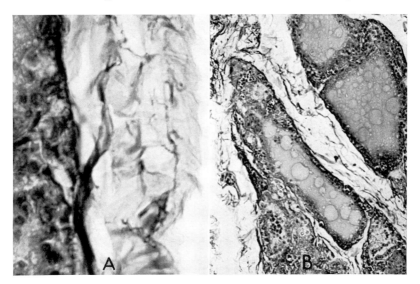

Fig. 14. Connective tissue of the capsule and the sustentacular tissue of the thyroid: *A*, outer layers of the capsule which have been teased apart showing the relation to the acini; *B*, interacinal tissue showing fine laminae lying directly against the cells (Weigert's elastic tissue stain).

laminated fibers interspersed with cells. These cells on section, appear spindleform, but when isolated are seen to be flat with ovoid nuclei (Fig. 13). The surface laminæ are covered with a more or less complete layer of such cells. This peritoneum-like structure accounts for the ease with which the gland glides about under the overlying structures on deglutition in the normal state, and also for the facility with which it reacts to irritative changes of the gland parenchyma in cases of acutely toxic goiters. The capsule contains some elastic fibers (Fig. 14), consequently the connective tissue takes on a glossy refraction like that of the peritoneum, indicating an elasticity, not possessed by ordinary connective tissue, which permits expansion to meet the changing requirements of the parenchyma.

From the capsule, sustentacula extend into the interior, dividing the gland more or less clearly into lobulations though they are less distinct than in the infant. From these heavier septa fiber bundles extend forming the walls of individual acini. These terminal fasciculi are very fine, being composed of thin bundles of reticular tissue in which there are a few spindle cells with long, narrow nuclei. In most places it forms a thin plane of tissue on which the acinal cells rest. This sustentacular tissue has much in common with the subendothelial connective tissue of the peritoneum. The upper lamellae are covered with cells containing large ovoid vesicular nuclei

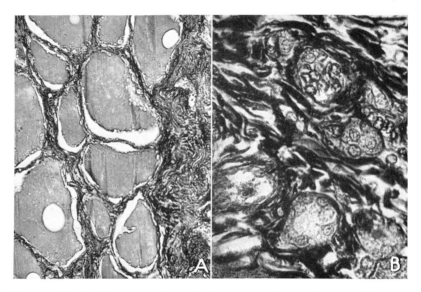

Fig. 15. Fibrosis of the normal thyroid in the aged: *A*, General increase of fibrous tissue about well preserved acini; *B*, Acinal epithelium degenerated and replaced by fibrous tissue (aniline blue stain). The fibrous tissue in both is nearly devoid of cells.

very similar to the endothelial cells of the peritoneum. They do not seem to differ from the capillary endothelium. Both may be composed of long sheets of protoplasm like the capillaries in the potential vessels of the peritoneum.

There is a considerable variation in individual cases and with the stain employed. With the regulation hematoxylin, eosin stain it may be scarcely visible (*A*, Fig. 15) but when Mallory's stain is used the fiber bundles stand out boldly (*B*, Fig. 15). It is obviously necessary therefore to know one's stain.

In children the connective tissue septa are more extensive than in the adult, but the interacinal connective tissue is not. In the aged the fibrous tissue is increased, as we shall see, but it is not uniformly distributed, sclerotic areas being interspersed with normal areas.

Blood Vessels. The blood reaches the gland through the superior and inferior thyroid arteries. They enter the capsule and are distributed throughout the septa. The walls of the arteries in the capsule are relatively thick, the muscle coat particularly, as compared to the other two coats (*A*, Fig. 16). Humps in the walls of the vessels have been described (*B*, Fig. 16).

The blood vessels, as noted in the gland of the infant, form an aston-

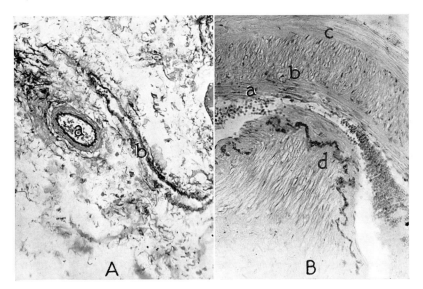

FIG. 16. Slide showing the comparative thickness of the walls of the arteries and veins, stressing the elastic tissue layer: *a*, artery, *b*, vein (Weigert's elastic tissue stain). *B*, Oblique section of an artery in the capsule: *a*, intima; *b*, muscular layer; *c*, fibrous layer; *d*, hump in the wall of the vessel partly occluding it.

ishingly rich capillary network. Their extent is more impressive when the native blood is retained in the gland than when there is injection of the vessel (*A*, Fig. 17). The vessels in the child equal in size the acini. In the adult they are less conspicuous though still large (*B*, Fig. 17). They lie in the connective tissue of the septa, there being only a single layer of connective tissue fibers between them and the acinal epithelium, and these are not in evidence unless the tissues are teased apart (*A*, Fig. 17). The vessels here have the same relation to the acinal cells that the vessels of the peritoneum do to the endothelium of the serosal surface.

The Veins. It is difficult to distinguish the veins from the arteries.

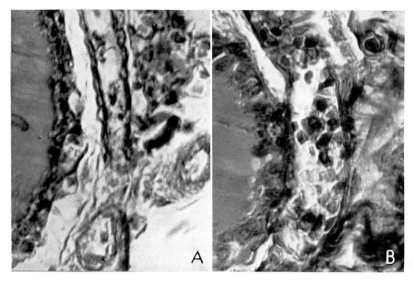

FIG. 17. Interacinal vessels distended with blood (trichrome II stain): *A*, partly teased apart showing the connective tissue between the vessel and acini; *B*, the vessel in direct contact with the acinal cells without apparent interposition of connective tissue.

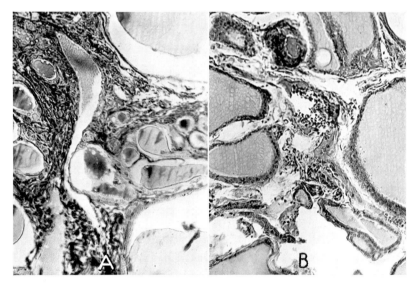

FIG. 18. Cross-section of thyroid veins. *A*, Longitudinal section of a vein in a fibrous septum. The wall of the vein suffuses with the surrounding fibrous tissue. *B*, Cross-section of veins at the juncture of several fibrous septa. The wall of the vein is suffused with the adjacent fibrous tissue.

The only difference is in the thickness of the walls; theoretically at least the veins lack a media. The veins as they near the periphery obtain much thicker coats (Fig. 18). When they leave the gland their structure is the same as that of any of the other veins leaving the viscera, e.g., the ovarian or mesenteric.

Lymph Vessels. The extent of the lymph channels has been variously estimated by different observers. The difficulty of demonstrating them is responsible for the discrepancies. Judging from silver preparations they are even more extensive than the capillaries. The question of their rela-

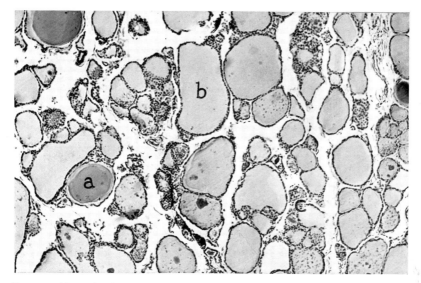

FIG. 19. Normal goiter showing acini of varying size and some basophilic colloid: *a,a*, acini containing basophilic colloid; *b,b*, acini containing normal colloid; *c,c*, many small acini, too numerous to make their origin from normal acini possible.

tion to the acinal cells has been much discussed. There is always a layer of connective tissue between the lymph sinus and the epithelium in well-stained specimens. When not demonstrable it should be ascribed to faulty technic, for one may be sure nature does not go to the trouble of supplying some with walls and of leaving others with none.

The Acini. The acini are closed sacs of round or ovoid form (Fig. 19) which vary in size from the microscopic to those visible to the naked eye.

The cells in the normal young adult may be said to be cuboidal with ovoid nuclei and faintly staining protoplasm (Fig. 20). They form a single uniform layer. The epithelium in different follicles is very dissimilar. However such a dissimilarity should excite a suspicion as to their normal state

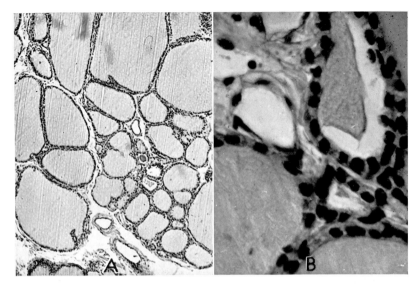

FIG. 20. Normal thyroid, M., age 28. Killed by blow on head. *A*, Acini of varying size lined by uniform epithelium and containing a uniform colloid. *B*, The epithelium is in the main cuboidal but some are flat. The colloid shows a variable degree of stainability.

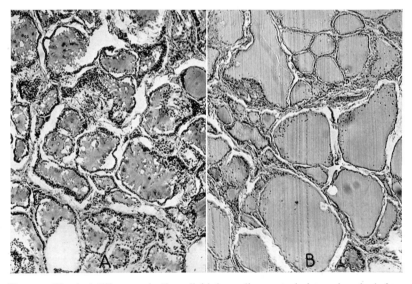

FIG. 21. Physical differences in the colloid depending on technic employed: *A*, frozen section. The colloid is vacuolated and several acini are empty. *B*, Formalin hardened, sectioned in paraffin. The colloid completely fills the acini. There are some exfoliated cells. (Autopsy specimen.)

even when encountered in apparently normal individuals. Cells of different type have been described but aside from difference in the dyes accepted by various cells in the same acinus there are no differences apparent by the simple technic of the surgical pathologist.

Much discussion has centered about the genesis and significance of the small acini or small groups of cells without lumina interspersed with those of usual size. These are most commonly seen in older persons, and though they apparently are in good health one cannot exclude the presence of an abortive attempt at compensatory hypertrophy, the first step toward an

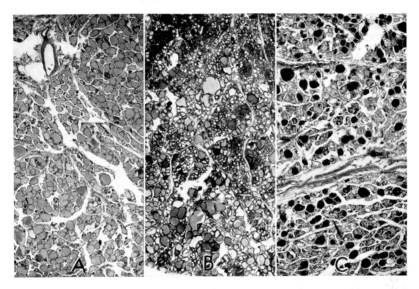

FIG. 22. Varying stainability of the colloid with different dyes: *A*, uniform staining with eosin, some are basophilic; *B*, varying staining with Mallory's aniline blue stain; *C*, marked contrast from light to very dark with phosphotungstic acid stain—some stain palely, some not at all.

abnormal state. The presence of basophilic colloid heightens this possibility.

The Colloid. The acini are filled with a uniform colloid. It varies in density, as gauged by the stainability, in different ages and likely in different physiologic states, and, of course, in different pathologic conditions. It is homogeneous and stains a uniform pale pink with eosin, exactly like red blood corpuscles.

Great variations are encountered in the normal state, due to the diverse technic employed in making the slides. Vacuoles are sometimes noted. These are uniformly present in frozen sections (*A*, Fig. 21), though absent in formalin hardened and paraffin imbedded sections from the same tissue (*B*, Fig. 21). Frozen sections show many empty follicles, the colloid having been shaken out during preparation.

A gland, the colloid of which stains a uniform normal pink, may show numerous variations with different dyes (Fig. 22). The significance of this is a matter of speculation.

Even more striking are the changes in staining characteristics in adjacent acini (Fig. 23). These changes are exceedingly complicated because

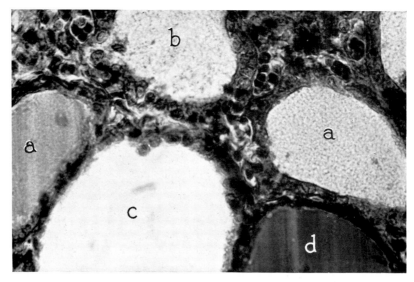

FIG. 23. Differences in stainability of adjacent acini in a patient who died some days following a brain injury: *a,a*, granular; *b*, palely staining granular; *c*, homogeneous but palely staining; *d*, deeply staining with the aniline. The epithelium in each is uniform. (Mallory's aniline blue stain.)

they are found in normal glands of patients who died of some disease, indicating a change in the colloid which escapes the usual routine technic.

Crenations of the colloid are sometimes mentioned. This likewise seems to be a matter of preparation (*A*, Fig. 24) but some tissues seem to show it more than others, hence it may have some significance if we but knew it. The crenated and vacuolated colloid acini may be situated alongside normal colloid (*B*, Fig. 24).

The variations above noted as occurring in normal goiters are so accepted because as such there was no demonstrable evidence of thyroid disease. Nevertheless, because of their constant association with obviously diseased states one feels that these changes are abnormal.

THE SENILE THYROID GLAND

Since the relation of certain goitrous states to the heart has now become generally recognized it is important to study the changes that occur in the supposedly normal thyroid gland with the advancing years.

That there are progressive changes in the thyroid gland in aging persons is a proposition that must be accepted in a general way. Naturally there cannot be a direct calendar relationship, such as that by which one determines the age of a horse by its teeth, because the progress of indi-

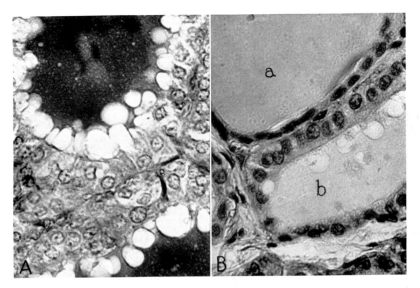

Fig. 24. Crenations of the colloid in follicles adjacent to those with normal colloid: *A*, marked crenation in tissue hardened in Muller's fluid. The colloid is basophilic, the cells cuboid; *B*, same tissue hardened in formalin: *a*, the colloid fills the acinus fully, the epithelium is flat; *b*, indications of crenation with columnar epithelium.

viduals toward senescence is variable. Just what shall be regarded as physiologic in old age it is hard to say. Like other sclerotic changes, notably of the arteries, those of the thyroid gland may be regarded as within the pale of the normal, being a part of a general constitutional process crystallized in the old saw "A man is as old as his arteries." The only method of approach is to see what sort of thyroid glands are possessed by supposedly normal individuals of different ages. My studies lead me to believe that some one some day will propose that instead of saying a man is as old as his arteries we shall say that a man is as old as the colloid in his thyroid gland.

Normal or not normal for a given age, a studious comparison of these glands with normal glands of early life reveals that they are obviously incapable of performing a normal thyroid function. Whether they are merely useless organs or whether they exert a deleterious influence it is impossible to say. It would be easy to say that after middle life, the thyroid having no longer any important function, follows the thymus into retirement.

The Capsule and Septa. Evidence of sclerosis may be found on gross inspection of the capsule indicated by the firmer consistency and whiter

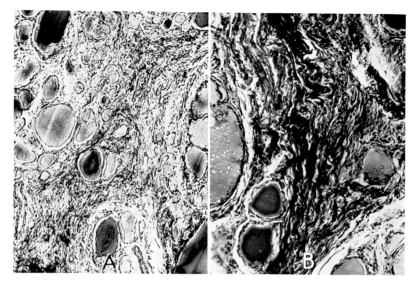

FIG. 25. Slide near the capsule of the thyroid gland of a woman aged 64: *A*, the parenchyma is largely replaced by wavy connective tissue. The acini are small and atrophic; *B*, the beginning of the septa are made up of heavy connective tissue (trichrome II stain).

color. On section certain areas may be fibrotic. The section may show distinct fibrous bands or scarred areas.

The slide of such tissues showing a simple sclerosis may be taken as a matter of course to be merely indicative of advancing years, but a connective tissue that is hyaloid in character as well as increased in amount (Fig. 25) suggests more than orderly retreat. The increase in fibrous tissue may be so great as to compress the enclosed acini, obliterating their lumen and giving the site the appearance of a carcinoma. In these the epithelium is deeply staining (see chapter on Tumors). The possibility should also be considered that the primary change may be in the acini and the

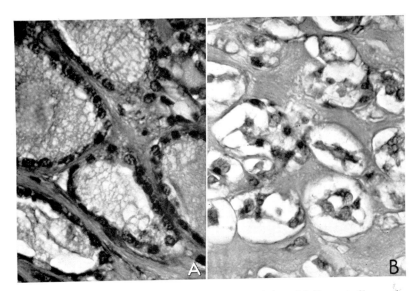

F<small>IG</small>. 26. Fibrosis of the thyroid with degeneration of the epithelium: *A*, fibrous tissue increase, epithelium partly degenerated, the colloid vacuolated; *B*, the acinal cells are completely degenerated, being attached to the walls only by slender process, and the colloid has disappeared.

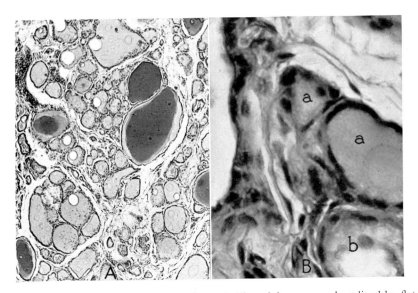

F<small>IG</small>. 27. Thyroid from a patient aged 70. *A*, The acini are everywhere lined by flat epithelium. The fibrous tissue is increased. *B, a,a*, The acinal epithelium is flat and in some areas, *b*, defective. The nuclei are deeply staining, due to advanced degeneration.

increase of connective tissue be merely a replacement process. This is indicated by the fact that the epithelium is in an advanced state of degeneration (Fig. 26).

The Acini. Cells of the acini are flat or irregular, obviously inactive,
and in some areas wholly defective. The cells are not exfoliated as one
sees in toxic goiters; they just flatten out and quit (Fig. 27). Occasionally
some acini, particularly the smaller ones in the spaces between the larger
ones, may show epithelial cells which resemble those in Hashimoto's
struma, granular protoplasm, that is sometimes even foamy. These areas

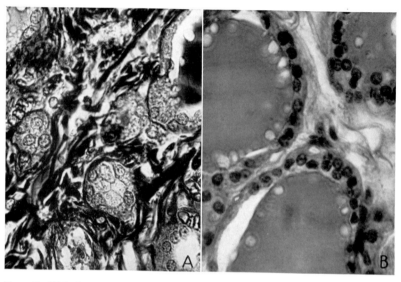

Fig. 28. Slide from a normal male, aged 70. *A*, Increase in fibrous tissue enclosing
islands of cells containing no lumina (Mallory's aniline blue). *B*, The colloid is deeply
staining, crenated and tends to retract. The epithelium is in part well preserved, in part
degenerated.

(Fig. 28), instead of representing compensatory hyperplasia as is generally believed, may be deleterious in their influence and calculated to
expedite our entrance to the happy hunting grounds.

The Colloid. Great variation in the amount and stainability of the
colloid is the chief fact of interest in the thyroid glands of aging persons.
The earlier changes are in the direction of decreasing acidophilic affinity
and advancing basophilic tinctorial reaction. Succeeding these are other
evidences of degeneration, vacuolation, granulation and shrinkage.

One not infrequently sees basophilic changes in young persons, even
in their teens, but this is not common until the fourth decade. These

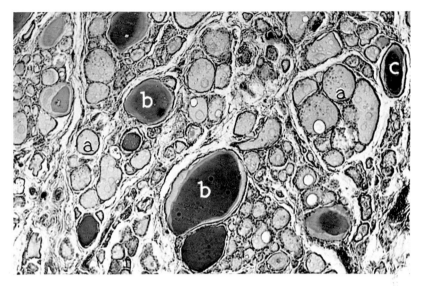

FIG. 29. Basophilic change in a normal thyroid gland. There is general fibrosis: *a,a*, acini with faintly staining acidophilic colloid; *b,b*, acini filled with basophilic colloid; *c*, basophilic colloid which has retracted (hematoxylin-eosin stain).

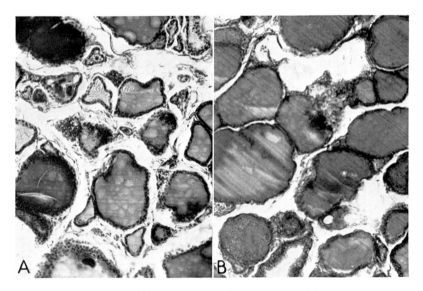

FIG. 30. Changes in a middle aged person showing a flat epithelium on a variously changed colloid. There is mottling in all the acini. *A*, The epithelium is retained, the colloid vacuolated (trichrome II stain). *B*, The epithelium is very flat, some areas absent (Mallory's aniline blue stain).

early changes are always associated with a flat and obviously inactive epithelium. Such acini we may assume are lost to the individual (Fig. 29). The variability of the structure of the colloid is shown by the use of special stain (Fig. 30).

The important point in the study of the colloid in normal thyroid glands is that it shows tinctorial changes identical with those seen in cardiotoxic goiters. This suggests that the thyroid need not attain goitrous dimensions in order to affect the heart. Possibly the thyroid gland, having brought us to the adult state, views us awhile and, becoming dissatisfied with us, lays low our hearts; the cruelty of creation thus giving way to the beneficence of death. Even the taxpayer may have a friend.

Literature

Anatomy. There are but two points in the anatomy of the thyroid of interest to the surgical pathologist: the formation of acini and the changes incident to advancing years.

Recent contributions to the structure of the thyroid gland have been illuminating but there are many points yet to be determined before the needs of the pathologist are fulfilled. The most interesting of these studies are the Born reconstructions. Unfortunately the method is too crude to permit the determination of cellular detail. Of these studies may be mentioned Rienhoff (*Arch. Surg.*, Dec. 1929, 19, 986–1036). By means of wax reconstruction models he has shown better than has been done heretofore that the thyroid is divided into parts. He decries the use of the term "lobules" but calls them bands, plates, bars, stalks and bulbs. Very well, we all have the same concepts, the only difference being in the choice of words. Let us compromise by saying the lobules by combining may form bands, plates, bars, stalks and bulbs. These bands, plates bars, stalks and bulbs, let it be added, are further subdivided into yet smaller ones, some of them containing only a few acini and are therefore microscopic in size. He says further that new acini are not formed. Wilson (*Anat. Rec.*, Nov. 1929, 37, 31–61) had previously made reconstructions. He comes to the conservative conclusion that by this method the origin of follicles is from cell masses and growth by fusion with follicles already present has been shown. This may be granted for the normal gland. However in the pathologic gland new acini are formed.

Valuable as reconstructions are the method is too crude to show cytologic detail. Structures this method does not show must not be declared to be nonexistent but that the models do not show them.

In contrast to these studies Zechel (*Surg., Gynec. and Obst.*, Feb. 1931, 52, 228–232) describes two types of intrafollicular cells: (*1*) One group remaining embryonal and awaiting development into follicles; (*2*) Those arising from the breaking up of follicles. He (*Ibid.*, Jan. 1932, 54, 1–5), in a later paper, discusses the cells of the parenchyma and finds the interfollicular cells most marked in regenerating goiter. These are the cells that I have been seeing in the so-called interstitial goiters. They resemble embryonal cells.

The question of the presence of normal changes with advancing years likewise caused the expression of opinion. Hinton (*Am. J. Surg.*, Feb. 1931, 269–279) found no relation in the changes to the different ages and McFarland and Robson (*Arch. Path.*, April 1929, 7, 628–639) are eloquent in denying any relationship though they did find some relation between fibrosis and chronic diseases. Both these papers are considered only with the calendar age without taking the previous state into account. Here, too, the conclusion should not include more than the minor premise. The methods employed do not show changes with advancing years. I believe a more extended study will bring different conclusions. Surely total thyroidectomies have demonstrated that there is a difference between the adolescent and the adult thyroid.

General pathologic changes certainly occur not directly associated with function. Pusch (*Arch. Path.*, Sept. 1932, 14, 353–359) was able to observe calcification in the walls of blood vessels in goiters. These were degenerative in nature and were more pronounced in advanced years. Hartoch (*Klin. Wchn.*, July 1932, 11, 1224–1225) was able to observe with the aid of the intravital microscope the exchange of colloid by direct observation. The significance of these observations is not apparent. Hellwig (*Arch. Path.*, March 1933, 15, 321–329) noted proliferation of epithelium of the acinal cells in rabbits after urine from pregnant women was injected in doing the Aschheim-Zondek test. The moral is rabbits should avoid the urine of pregnant women.

Not infrequently apparently newly formed acini are found in glands of old people. The colloid is seldom normal and it may be possible these acini develop in response to the degenerating connective tissue. This is not the whole explanation because in rare cases patients with goiters present such structures and mild symptoms of hyperplastic toxicity. These therefore cannot all be placed in the same category. Dogliotti and Nizzi Nuti (*Endocrinology*, May-June 1935, 19, 289–292) published a paper on this phase and faithfully reproduce the unstable nature of the colloid.

Lymphatics. Chouke, Whitehead and Parker (*Surg., Gynec. and Obst.*, June 1932, 54, 865–871) find no relation between the lymphatics of the thymus and thyroid. These vessels seem to emerge from the superficial surface of the thyroid and enter nearby lymph nodes and thence to the large trunks. Williamson and Pearse (*Brit. J. Surg.*, Jan. 1930, 17, 529–550) on the other hand find a direct connection forming between the two a closed system. These authors make the further observation that some of the cysts found in the thyroid gland are but dilated lymph spaces. This agrees with my observations. This is an unusually fine research and is worthy of careful examination. Rienhoff (*Arch. Surg.*, Nov. 1931, 23, 783) has been astonishingly successful in the demonstration of the lymph plexuses about the acini of the dog. These injection pictures are much more complete (in the dog) than is possible to demonstrate in the human by the silver method.

CHAPTER III

General Pathology of Goiter

THE general laws governing pathologic processes have been too largely ignored in the study of the thyroid gland. Certain changes mean a certain thing in all pathology and require a certain time to develop. The literature is burdened with statements that on the face of them are impossible, implying changes that cannot possibly have taken place in the time specified. Unfortunately for the surgeon these detailed facts cannot be acquired by looking over the shoulder of the pathologist; the price is the smell of formalin, xylol and balsam.

It is the purpose of this chapter to correlate, as far as possible, the changes which occur in the thyroid with the general laws of pathology. These being recognized, it is unnecessary to refute individually and in detail some of the things written about and even accepted which most certainly never happened.

It is necessary to recognize in the outset that the changes in the thyroid, due partly to disease, partly to changes incident to advancing years, are so complicated that one requires a different concept in many respects than that applicable to the pathology of other organs. Nevertheless, there are the fundamental processes of inflammation and fibrosis and certain epithelial changes that cannot escape the general laws governing all tissues. Furthermore, it is the purpose of this chapter to align certain processes more or less specific to the thyroid gland with those of general pathology. This, it is hoped, will serve as a sort of glossary, making comparison easier in the discussions to be presented in the special chapters to follow.

The thyroid gland, broadly speaking, is made up of three components, as considered in the chapter on normal morphology, namely, the connective tissue, the acinal epithelium and the colloid. The various changes that occur in these three groups of tissues are discussed separately though of course the changes are more or less simultaneous and interdependent. Thus connective tissue changes, proliferative and degenerative, are discussed without relation to other parts of the gland. Cells of varying forms, flat, cuboidal or columnar, and their arrangement are discussed without relation to the connective tissue. Changes in the colloid, pale, liquid, basophilic and so forth, are considered without relation to the epithelium and the connective tissue. It is hoped that such a plan will

42

make it possible to use the unit changes in any combination to descriptively report what one finds in the various diseases discussed in subsequent chapters irrespective of the age of the individual, of the kind of goiter we have diagnosed in the clinic, and even if there is no evidence of a goiter at all.

Generally speaking, the only knowledge the surgeon can use is that based on what he himself can visualize. What he sees in the gross must bring to his mind's eye what the microscope will show him. For instance, a certain type of gland will at the operating table conjure up for him the picture a microscopic study will reveal: for example, sparse connective tissue, papillary epithelium, pale colloid; Basedow's disease. These histologic details are simple enough for him to see under the microscope and are sufficient to aid in placing that particular goiter in its proper group while he still has his gloves on.

Detail that he never sees, accessible only to some one particular individual who has developed a special laboratory technic, is of no use to him regardless of its biologic interest or its possible theoretic importance. Usually such knowledge is purely academic since the structures found bear no relation to the disease processes as we know them today. I have in mind the various kinds of cells described in normal acini. Usually such structures are seen by only one investigator, or, if several see them, there is a disagreement as to their import. Generally speaking, until pathologists are agreed upon the meaning of structural variation, the surgeon will do well to look on it as parlor knowledge and to eschew it in his clinical thinking. For instance as we used to look on stomata as essential integrals in our concepts of inflammation and absorption, we now know they are artefacts and the processes of inflammation and absorption go on as before.

Yet I am obliged to confess that much of what is here presented will appear "parlor knowledge" to many readers. However, though some of it must be tentatively presented, I believe that examination of a sufficient number of cases will justify me imparting my conclusions here. This remark applies particularly to the histochemical changes in the colloid. Be this as it may, any one accepting my views does so at his own peril. The ideas are my own.

One must ask himself at the outset, how does a goiter get that way? I mean in an anatomic, not in an etiologic sense. That is, what makes the thyroid gland get big? Obviously, it being made up of acini, the explanation is confined to one or both of two alternatives: the old acini get bigger, or new acini are formed. It is necessary to keep these facts in mind in considering the various structures that go to make up a goiter.

The general pathologic changes which admit of abstract discussion may be listed as follows:

   I. Changes in the Connective Tissue
      Hyperplasia of Connective Tissue
         Replacement
         Reactive
      Fibrinous Changes in the Connective Tissue
      Degeneration of Connective Tissue
         Hyaline
         Calcareous
      Hyperplasia of the Elastic Fibers

  II. Epithelium
      Hypertrophy of the Acinal Epithelium
      Hyperplasia of the Acinal Epithelium (Formation of Bosselations)
      Atrophy
      Desquamation

 III. Colloid
      Acidophile
      Basophile
      Vacuolated
      Rarefied
      Dense

  IV. Degenerative Changes Which Affect the Constitution
      The Cardiotoxic Goiter
      Myxedema

The above classification obviously includes only those changes common more or less to all goiters. Those changes which apply to only one type of goiter may most conveniently be considered in the discussion of those goiters in which that particular change is found.

CONNECTIVE TISSUE

The connective tissue in goiters may undergo one of two changes, it may increase in amount—a hyperplasia, or it may undergo one or other of the degenerative changes as observed in general pathology. An increase in amount may be due to a reactive state or to replacement after degeneration of the parenchyma. Only as the end result of inflammatory process can one think of a purposive hyperplasia, that developing in parenchymal degeneration is of different import.

In degenerative processes the connective tissue suffers, as well as the parenchyma, from the disturbances in nutrition or those due to involutional processes. The study of the connective tissue in goiters is therefore both a quantitative as well as a qualitative one. The study of the connective tissue changes in goiters must be based on a study in tinctorial chemistry rather than on morphology. This is necessary because in very toxic goiters the only change to be noted is a tinctorial one. The same is true in replacement and degenerative tissues.

Hyperplasia of Connective Tissue. An active increase in the normal amount of connective tissue suggests one of the two possibilities noted

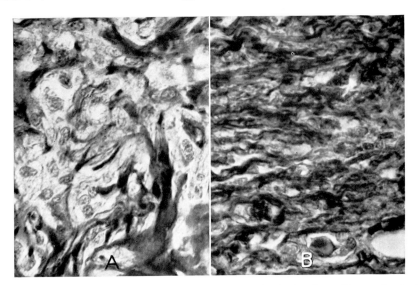

Fig. 31. Replacement fibrosis in a degenerating gland: *A*, all semblance of acinal formation has been lost; interspersed by fibrous tissue; *B*, advanced stage of fibrosis, only a few acini and cells are preserved at the lower part (Mallory's aniline blue).

above; namely as a replacement process in parenchymatous degeneration or as the result of an inflammatory process.

Increase in connective tissue incident to degeneration in the parenchyma incident to disease; or due to advancing years is purely a replacement process. Degenerated parenchyma tends to become supplanted by connective tissue as is true of disease of any other organ following death of tissue. Such processes usually carry a cognomen indicative of an inflammatory process but there is no justification for this. It is rather a hyperplasia incident to the irritation of the ailing parenchyma. Even calling it a hyperplasia is assuming much since often it is but a swelling from a pure degeneration.

This type of connective tissue is characterized by the indistinct out-line of the individual fibers and by the sparsity of the nuclei which stain but faintly. The fibrils stain with acid dyes but faintly and unequally but stain deeply with aniline blue (Fig. 31).

It is impossible to say how long such tissue is in forming but it is at least many months, usually years, as one may judge from the general history of the goiter.

The only true hyperplasia of the connective tissue in the thyroid gland is found as the end result of a defensive reaction; that is, a thy-

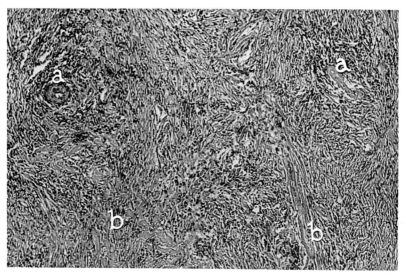

FIG. 32. Nonsuppurative thyroiditis of some eight week's duration: *a,a*, small blood vessels surrounded by round cell infiltration; *b,b*, interlacing bundles of fibrous tissue containing many ovoid deeply staining nuclei. The connective tissue appears yellowish red when stained with van Gieson's.

roiditis. This is seen most typically in nonsuppurative thyroiditis (Fig. 32) and in Riedel's struma. The latter is characterized by heavy keloid-like bundles (Fig. 33). In this condition the connective tissue stains deeply with acid dyes, most typically with van Gieson's stain. Of course, during the terminal stages of acute inflammations the cells are larger, less spindleform, the protoplasm more abundant and the fibers stain less intensely with specific dyes.

Here also it is sometimes of interest to estimate the probable duration of the process. The formation of adult fibrous tissue following a reactive process is a matter of months. In wound healing under ideal conditions, in the absence of all reactive phenomena it takes at least three weeks. Even at this time the cells are still ovoid indicating a recent vintage.

Fibrinoid Changes in the Connective Tissue. The study of the connective tissue of the thyroid capsule, I am obliged to confess, is the result of my studies in inflammation in general and of peritonitis in particular. I venture to include it here because it explains the phenomena of the adherent goiter in cases of extreme thyroid toxicity as seen notably in Graves' disease.

I mean by fibrinous change, the tinctorial changes which occur in the connective tissue when subjected to irritation. What makes the very

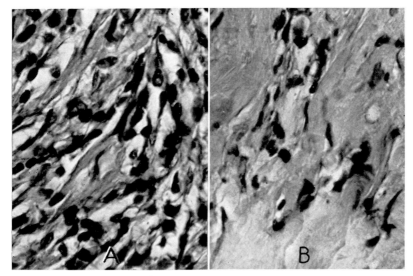

Fig. 33. Riedel's struma of some months' duration: *A*, early stage in which there is extensive fibrosis; newly formed fiber bundles interspersed with nuclei of many forms and sizes; *B*, heavy bundles of keloid-like fibers with few irregular nuclei. The fiber bundles stain intensely with van Gieson's.

toxic goiter become immobile under the ribbon muscles is a question which must have come to the mind of every surgeon while attempting the removal of a very toxic goiter. The same question plagues him when confronted with a gland as friable as granulation tissue. Granulation tissue is friable, as is well known, because the fibrin has not yet formed connective tissue. In a friable goiter the process is reversed. It was once adult connective tissue but, as the result of irritation of the thyroid parenchyma, it has returned to a previous state approaching fibrin. Any surgeon who has inadvertently torn an inflamed gut while separating adhesions has met this same process. The normal gut wall has, due to irritation, become as friable as wet blotting paper so that a slight pressure with the finger suffices to rupture it.

The connective tissue of the friable goiter reacts to dyes exactly as does the fibrinous connective tissue in exuberant granulation tissue, or the gut wall about an abscess. In other words the connective tissue has regressed toward the embryonal stage (Fig. 34). This regressive change is evinced by the fact that the connective tissue no longer accepts the connective tissue stain in a typical manner but approaches the tinctorial reaction of fibrin. It stains reddish brown with eosin and very indiffer-

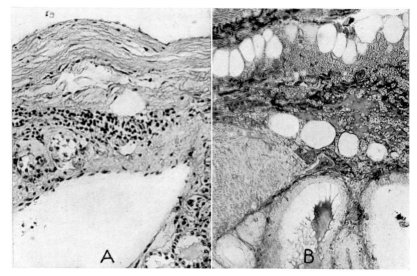

FIG. 34. Fibrinoid connective tissue in toxic goiter: *A*, capsule, the connective tissue of which stains a faint brown with van Gieson's stain; round cell infiltration beneath; *B*, fiber bundles staining a dirty blue with Mallory's aniline blue; below several acini the cells of which stain but faintly.

erently with van Gieson's stain. That is to say it responds by a refusal of the fibers to take the fuchsin stain with a normal bright red color and stains instead a dirty brown. Inasmuch as it refuses the blue stain in Weigert's stain it is something less than true fibrin, hence the term "fibrinoid."

Just what causes the connective tissue in very toxic goiters thus to lose its affinity for acid dyes and tend to regress toward the fibrin stage is not known. We must assume that the toxicity of the acinal epithelium exerts much the same influence on the connective tissue as does the inflammatory exudate in inflammation. The result is the capsule of the thyroid gland becomes adherent to the overlying structures. The changes are identical with those of an aseptic peritonitis. In this condition, like the changes in connective tissue inflammation, it is capable of returning to normal when the irritation is removed. This allows the previously fixed goiter to again become movable. This is important for the wise surgeon sometimes elects to defer operation until the gland becomes movable, indicating that the height of friability has passed, making the operation safer and the technic easier. After this state subsides the adhesion releases and the separation of the gland from the surrounding tissue becomes easy.

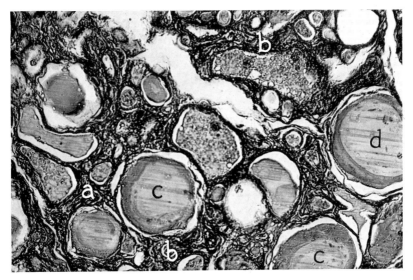

FIG. 35. Replacement fibrosis in an old colloid goiter: *a*, increase in fibrous tissue; *b,b*, atrophic acini; *c,c*, acini with basophilic colloid, epithelium wholly atrophic; *d* acinus in which the colloid is degenerated, the epithelium lost.

Degenerative Changes in Connective Tissue. In the foregoing paragraphs changes are considered which imply some active or reactive response on the part of the connective tissue. The connective tissue has done something on its own account. Here we have to do with connective tissue which has suffered passively from its environment. Here also the connective tissue becomes friable so that if the capsule is cut the gland parenchyma oozes out like very friable exuberant granulation tissue. Unlike the friability discussed in the preceding section, this tissue never again returns to normal.

In certain types of long existing goiters, notably the nodulated colloid, the fibers degenerate. The connective tissue is characterized by a reduced affinity for the usual acid dyes (Fig. 35), or for any other dye for that matter. One may even postulate the general principle that any tissue that refuses all dyes has already died.

The connective tissue degeneration found in goiter does not respond tinctorially like similar changes in other organs. One of the commonest changes of the connective tissue resembles hyaline degeneration in that it becomes glassy and reacts to certain specific stains, such as a phospho-tungstic acid, but not typically, refusing all acid stains or even becomes basophilic. Usually there are no cells or at most only ovoid palely stain-ing ones. The use of the term "hyaline" is used as a group term without an attempt to designate the exact changes which are unknown to me. This type of degeneration is seen most commonly in old nodular goiters and in the normal glands of old persons.

The connective tissue in old fetal adenomas undergoes a different change. One might call it mucinous save that it refuses to react to specific dyes. In fact it refuses any dye but tends to liquefy resulting in a cystic cavity.

Infiltration with lime salts, calcareous infiltration, may be regarded as the end stage of all degenerations, nature's requiem as it were.

However, the deposit of calcium does not confine itself to the con-nective tissue since the epithelium and colloid tissue are likewise infil-trated, though the connective tissue is most extensively involved.

Insignificant therefore as calcareous infiltration is in its pathologic physiologic relations, to the surgeon it may be important. When the calcareous deposit cements the capsule of the gland to adjacent struc-tures, such as the trachea, particularly to a large vein, it becomes of technical importance, especially in large substernal goiters.

There is said to be changes in the elastic tissue resulting in an in-crease in certain types of goiter. Unfortunately the elastic dyes are un-certain in my hands and so far as I can see one may conclude that, if he is so disposed, this tissue is increased. At any rate such increase, if it be present, is of unknown significance.

CHANGES IN THE EPITHELIUM

Although a great variety of changes may occur in the epithelium, hyperplasia, atrophy and degeneration are of chief importance in the pathology of the thyroid gland. Tinctorial changes occur in the epi-thelium but the significance is not understood. The most constant of these that has come to my notice is that in the use of the trichrome stain some of the acinal nuclei stain blue, others red. These differences in the cells are confined to old degenerated goiters.

Much liberty has been taken by imputing potentialities to certain changes or states of the acinal epithelium. The term "resting" has been applied to flat epithelium implying that it is only temporarily quiescent. That these same cells may become cuboid or manifest other evidence of renewed activity at a later date cannot of course be demonstrated. We cannot put it back and look at it again some other time. Flat epithelium as seen in the thyroid gland is flat epithelium. That it is capable of going to work again has not been satisfactorily substantiated. We must admit that it may recrudesce but if and when it does, it becomes pathologic.

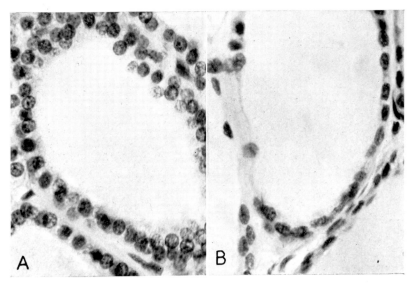

Fig. 36. Hyperplasia of the acinal epithelium: *A*, hypertrophy of the acinal epithelium which involved only a few acini in certain areas of the goiter; *B*, nearly all the goiter was made up of flat epithelium, in some areas nearly wholly atrophic.

That a flat epithelium should resume its normal function seems improbable because of associated changes, notably the development of numerous small acini and the changes in the chemical reaction of the colloid. Considering our present knowledge, therefore, atrophic seems a more accurate term than "resting."

In discussing the increased activity of acinal epithelium it is necessary to apply the terms "hypertrophy" and "hyperplasia" as used in general pathology.

Hypertrophy of the Acinal Epithelium. As generally used this term implies an increase in size of the acinal cells (Fig. 36). We cannot say by looking at a cell that it has undergone enlargement but if a colloid goiter becomes toxic and knowing that the acinal epithelium in the colloid is flat, we find it cuboidal or columnar in a toxic goiter, we may infer that the flat epithelium has become abnormally active. At any rate something has happened to produce thyroid toxicity. Perhaps one might say the resting stage has been converted into an active one. If so the activity has become pathologic. This simple change is seen only in early stages of toxic goiter and chiefly in young subjects. It seldom exists without associated hyperplasia.

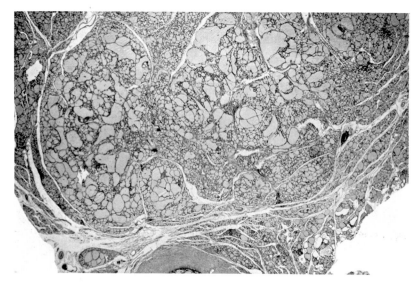

FIG. 37. Formation of a nodule in a nontoxic goiter. Many new acini are found in the walls of the old ones and the result is a gradual expansion of a certain area of gland. The increase in size is due to the large number of new acini and but in a minor degree to the increase in size of the old acini.

Hyperplasia of the Acinal Epithelium. In contradistinction to the above, we mean by hyperplasia an increase in the number of the cells of the acini. The two situations in which a numerical increase of cells is unmistakable are in the formation of new acini, in the spaces between old acini or in their walls as in nodular colloid goiter (Fig. 37), and in the formation of many small acini some of which have papillary excrescences which project into the lumina of acini as exemplified in the goiters of children with exophthalmos (Fig. 38). These small excrescences, though attended by eye signs, differ materially from the cell hyperplasia as observed in true Basedow's disease (Fig. 39). This difference is shown further in that in the bases of many of them new acini are forming.

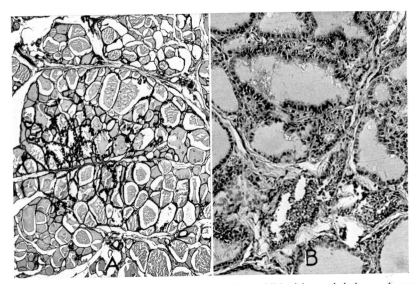

FIG. 38. Hyperplasia of the acinal epithelium in a child with exophthalmos: *A*, very small excrescences here and there protruding into the lumina of the acini; *B*, high power of same; lumina formation in the bases of some of them. The papillations are low but numerous.

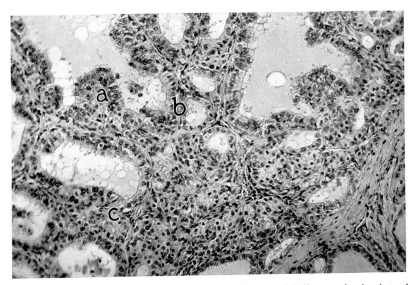

FIG. 39. Basedow's disease: *a*, papules of hyperplastic epithelium projecting into the acini; *b*, newly formed acini containing but little colloid and that vacuolated and palely staining; *c*, masses without lumina but the cells stain like those of the newly formed acini.

When a goiter increases in size, one or both of two things may befall, either the colloid in the old acini is augmented in volume or new acini are formed as noted above. In many cases both these factors are operative. In fact, save in the simple goiters of childhood and adolescence and some acutely toxic ones, goiter is nearly always associated with hyperplasia of the acinal epithelium as well as the increase of colloid.

We need now to inquire just how these two agencies act to produce augmentation in volume. Generally speaking the diffuse and nodular colloid goiters involve a different process from the acutely toxic goiters.

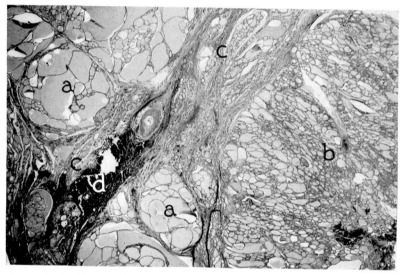

Fig. 40. Old nodular colloid: *a,a,* very large acini; *b,* large active nodule—the one that is active is causing increase in the size of the goiter; *c,c,* areas of gland not in active growth and have been compressed, forming a pseudo capsule; *d,* area of hemorrhage.

The normal gland is divided into regions by fibrous tissue septa and when a nodular goiter forms, these spaces which are formed by fibrous tissue, are distended as the acini increase in volume and a spheroidal lump forms.

In simple uniform goiters of adolescence all the acini contribute to the increase in the size of the gland by increasing their colloid content equally. The result is an equitable increase of the gland in all its parts. Though the connective tissue-confined acini form spheroidal areas there are no bosselations because all acini throughout the whole gland are enlarged to a like degree. Therefore, the gland remains symmetrically enlarged as one sees chiefly in adolescents. As bosselations form certain areas partake more than others in the formation of new acini. Why this is so we do not know. However, there results a compression of those acini not engaged in hyperplasia and they come to form a sort of capsule for the nodule (Fig. 40).

As these nodular colloids become toxic a more active process is added. The newly formed acini instead of being lined by flat epithelium (*A*, Fig. 41) become cuboidal, declaring a greater activity (*B*, Fig. 41). Such changes are usually confined to small areas while the greater part of the goiter retains the old colloid structure.

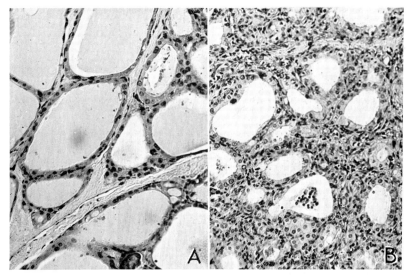

FIG. 41. Variation in different areas in an acutely toxic goiter: *A*, area showing simple colloid structure, large acini with uniform pale colloid; *B*, acini lined with columnar cells, the colloid stainless or granular. The cells stain equally. There is an absence of papule formation.

In the process just discussed there may be a question as to whether the process should be classed as hyperplasia, comprising compensatory formation of new acini, or as adenomas. This problem will be further discussed in the chapters on nodular goiters.

In the acutely toxic goiters the problem is a different one. Here the actual cell increase forms more or less of the bulk of the gland. Commonly here too a considerable part of the goiter is made up of simple dilated acini filled with uniform colloid, while a minor part is made up of acini containing active cells. It is sometimes confusing to observe that goiters with but small areas of obvious activity may be as toxic as those made up almost entirely of cell masses. However, the most viciously toxic cases are made up almost entirely of acini containing little colloid (*A*, Fig. 42) or none at all (*B*, Fig. 42). These very cellular goiters are usually relatively small, uniform and hard.

We are possessed of a limited amount of knowledge as to why colloid forms in thyroids of children. The collection of colloid in these simple goiters can well be considered a chemical problem involving, say, the lack of iodine. Why new acini form, why any sort of cellular hyperplasia is set in motion is beyond us. Our poverty of knowledge is evident when we invoke the mysterious activity of the parasympathetic system. When

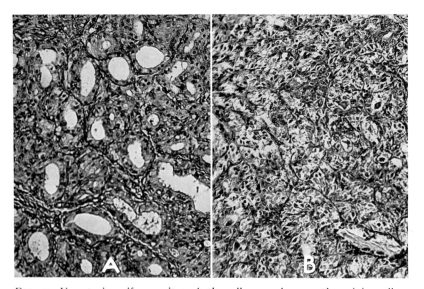

F IG. 42. Very toxic uniform goiter: *A*, the cells are columnar, the acini small, containing but little stainless colloid; *B*, the entire area is made up of cells without acini. Some of the cells show beginning degeneration as manifest by pale protoplasm and tendency to loosen from their bases.

new acini begin to form the acinal epithelium is usually flat, apparently inactive, the colloid pale or basophilic in spots. One might think that the epithelium proliferates because it is irritated by abnormal colloid without any thought of serving the host by a compensatory action. In acutely toxic goiters all acini, new and old, may have cuboidal or higher epithelium. It is these new acini which give us the index to toxicity. The colloid is always abnormal but which is hen and which is egg we can only surmise.

Atrophy of the Acinal Epithelium. As noted before it is difficult to distinguish the inactive or "resting" epithelium from actual atrophy. So long as the acinus contains an acidophilic colloid we may designate it by a complimentary cognomen but once the colloid becomes basophilic the day of usefulness of the acinal epithelium is definitely at an end. We encounter a new difficulty in determining what is the atrophy of old age and what is disease. Perhaps they are synonymous. Possibly when we acquire an acinus with atrophic epithelium we have made a step toward old age.

In thyroid glands of the aged and in old goiters the epithelium is usually flat. Usually there is associated fibrous tissue hyperplasia (*A*,

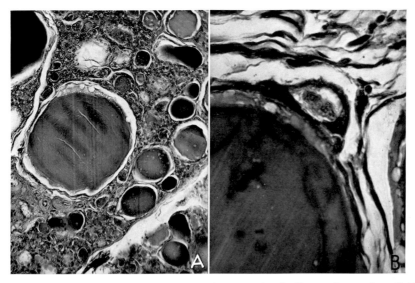

Fig. 43. Atrophic acinal epithelium: *A*, increase of pale fibrous tissue, the colloid uniform or vacuolated, the acinal epithelium defective; *B*, acini basophilic for the most part; the epithelium has wholly disappeared. The connective tissue is increased (Mallory's aniline blue).

Fig. 43). The epithelium is not only flat but may be actually defective. The acini may be small almost to the point of disappearance, may contain only a stainless colloid but most of the acini contain a basophilic colloid (*B*, Fig. 43). Such pictures as this certainly represent tissue of no possible use to the patient.

Degeneration of the Epithelium. In contradistinction to atrophy, degeneration is a condition in which an otherwise viable cell loses its life for some reason or other indicative of a more rapid process. Degeneration of acinal epithelium is usually secondary to a generally reduced nutritional state.

Thus old degenerating goiters are marked by the formation of much fibrous tissue and slow degeneration of cells is the natural result. The nuclei can be said to have lost their capacity to stain, the borders of the cells are frayed (Fig. 44). These changes may occur without there being an atrophy implying thereby that their demise is due to some extraneous factor. In this type the cells do not lose their place in their regular order about the lumen of the acini.

In more extensive degenerations cells are cast off and lie free in the colloid. This is properly called a desquamation and indicates an acute

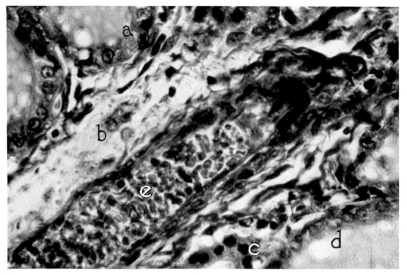

FIG. 44. Degeneration of acinal epithelium in an old colloid goiter: *a*, nuclei lost and protoplasm granular; *b*, faintly staining fibrous tissue; *c*, pyknotic cells; *d*, colloid and connective tissue faintly staining; *e*, large blood vessel containing blood.

process involving the whole gland, and is generally expressive of an excessively toxic state, whether it be an old degenerated colloid or a Basedow (Fig. 45). In hyperacute toxic goiters particularly cells may be cast off completely leaving whole acini bare of cells. This is what one sometimes sees in cases which run a fatal course in a few weeks. Generally speaking when desquamation is seen in a slide one may know that the patient has met a sudden end from goiter.

COLLOID

Normal colloid is uniform, fills the acinus completely and stains pale pink with eosin, the color being exactly that of red corpuscles.

Possible pathologic changes in the colloid have been very little studied. Thin, thick and vacuolated have been the chief mutations noted. However, when studied by more complicated dyes, a great variety of changes are found in the colloid. Such changes must have a meaning even though at present we cannot interpret them.

Thin Colloid. In the preceding chapter it was noted that normal colloid stains palely with eosin. When the stain is less intense than normal the colloid is said to be thin (*A*, Fig. 46). When nothing stains, the acini are said to be empty. If that be so, what keeps them distended? It must

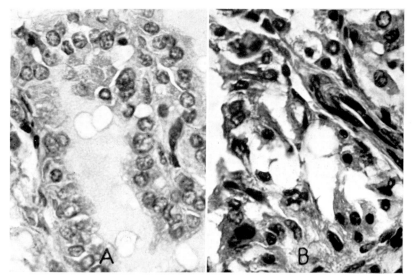

FIG. 45. Degenerating acutely toxic goiter: *A*, the nuclei are variously staining, some wholly degenerated, the colloid is vacuolated and degenerated; *B*, the acinal cells are illy shaped and variously degenerated, exfoliated. The colloid has all but disappeared.

be air pressure or something. As a matter of fact no such assumption is needed for when "empty" acini are stained with dyes other than eosin, the presence of colloid or something else is shown. Empty acini, unless the colloid has fallen out in the preparation of the slide, do not exist. Empty acini are common in formalin-hardened tissue cut in frozen sections. By penciling one may shake out the colloid of most acini. A pale staining colloid is usually associated with cellular hyperplasia, therefore it is most marked in very toxic goiters and is to a degree a measure of toxicity.

Thick Colloid. Thick colloid, in contradistinction to the preceding, is indicated when the staining with eosin is more intense than in the normal (*B*, Fig. 46). It is commonly present in old colloid goiters, particularly when there is degeneration of the connective tissue. One may speculate whether or not the colloid is thick because the state of the connective tissue slows absorption. At any rate a deeply eosin-staining colloid represents the last stage of usefulness.

Basophilic. The basophilic colloid described in the preceding section is found in all sorts of glands, apparently normal and in simple colloid glands in even young persons. This degeneration may not stain with hematoxylin and is demonstrated only with special stains. This may be designated merely thick colloid. By basophilic colloid we mean that con-

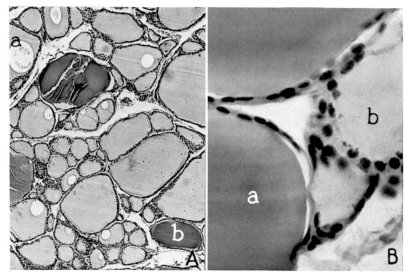

FIG. 46. Variable colloid in a normal gland: *A*, variously staining colloid, *a*, vacuolated; *b*, slightly basophilic in acini lined by normal cells; *B*, *a*, basophilic colloid in acini lined by atrophic cells; *b*, acini palely staining with all dyes.

dition in which the colloid stains a blue with the hematoxylin (Fig. 47). This form of colloid is pathologic and is associated with an atrophic and degenerated epithelium. Deeply staining acini are commonly associated with those staining palely (Fig. 47).

On the whole the abnormal staining of the colloid is more pronounced in old goiters which are the seat of degenerations and in goiters associated with heart failure. This suggests the possibility that such colloid represents a substance which affects adversely the heart function. One gets the impression that those acini which contain basophilic colloid are permanently functionless.

Vacuolated. Vacuoles are found in the colloid in all sorts of conditions the significance of which is not understood (Fig. 48). The change consists of open spaces in the colloid. The cavities may be small or large, single or multiple.

Serrated. The colloid is said to be serrated when there are regular vacuoles present about the border of the colloid so that there is contact with the acinal epithelium by tooth-like processes (Fig. 48).

Granular. In some cases the colloid is granular, deeper staining particles being intermingled with lighter ones. This structure is the rule

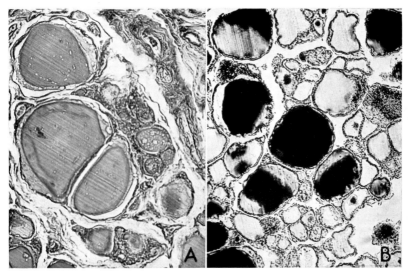

FIG. 47. Normal thyroid, F., aged 46. *A*, Colloid moderately basophilic with hematoxylin-eosin stain. *B*, some acini deeply staining; others not at all with phosphotungstic acid stain. The epithelium is flat, faintly staining and obviously quite incapable of function.

in frozen section. Some cases however are so constructed while others are uniform.

EFFECT OF THE GOITER ON THE CONSTITUTION

Having taken a cursory look at the various changes which take place in the thyroid gland there is yet a thought to be given as to the various influences these changes may have on the constitution. We have long known that hyperplasia spelled thyrotoxicosis, finding its superlative degree in exophthalmic goiter. We are beginning to realize that a degenerated goiter likewise finds expression in the well being of the individual. That is to say there is a toxicity of degeneration as well as a toxicity of hyperplasia. That degeneration ultimately finds expression as a goiter heart is now generally recognized but that degeneration may cause a variety of disturbances before the heart is noticeably affected has not been recognized. These disturbances may find expression in both nutritional and nervous manifestations. These are usually assumed to be due to cellular hyperplasia and not finding such changes in the slide confusion is caused. The anatomic evidence of toxicity of degeneration must be sought in the tinctorial changes in the colloid and not in hyperplasia

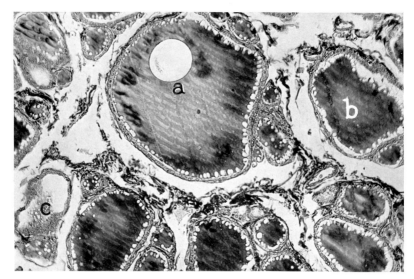

Fig. 48. Vacuolated and serrated colloid which is in part basophilic: *a*, large vacuole in an acinus partly basophilic; *b*, serrated colloid, also basophilic; *c*, acinus partly filled with granular colloid, the epithelium of which has degenerated.

of the epithelium. Only by this means can the clinical and the pathologic be harmonized.

Operations are done chiefly because the goiter is injuring the patient by making her nervous and causing loss of weight; that is, because the goiter is toxic. The operator removes as much of the toxin-producing gland as he dares. Less commonly operations are done because the goiter is causing pressure, or because the enlargement is unsightly. All these objects are attained by removing a part of the gland.

The fact is generally overlooked that the part of the gland left behind may cause a late cardiac failure without there ever having been a renewed nervousness or loss of weight. Of what use that part of the gland we ordinarily leave behind is should be studied anew. There may be some difference of opinion whether or not a hyperplastic toxic gland may return to normal, therefore a technical excuse for leaving a part. This is certainly true in children. In the degenerative toxic gland, on the other hand, there is no doubt but the entire gland is totally and permanently worse than useless. The only excuse for leaving a part of such a gland is wholly a technical one.

It now has been abundantly demonstrated that in the adult there is no limit to the amount of gland that can safely be removed. Generally speaking, therefore, we are obligated to remove all that part of the gland which is capable of future mischief.

The study of the pathology of goiters has progressed but little beyond general principles but it is really a study of individuals. The variations in individual cases are so great that each patient must be regarded as a concrete problem in pathology. Generalizations must come last, not first.

Literature

The fundamental factor of interest to the surgeon is the nature of the goitrous disease. Is the noise due to a player piano gone wrong or is it the result of a poor pianist playing on a good instrument? —if the former, a good mechanic may hope to restore harmony, if the latter, he is helpless. With more and more complete operations the probability increases that goiter is a disease of the thyroid gland and that the surgeon is justified in increasing his energies in the effort to solve the problem.

The recent paper by Boothby (*Arch. Int. Med.*, July 1934, 56, 136–206) in so far as a surgeon can hope to comprehend it indicates that there are certain substances that play a primary rôle. The more one pays attention to the interrelation between pituitary and thyroid the more does it seem likely that these two organs are responsible for the disturbances. This tends to eliminate the sympathetic nervous system as a causative factor in the production of goitrous diseases. Of course the general constitutional condition, including the nervous system, has an influence in determining the manifestations of the disease just as it does the diseases of many other organs. At any rate as the problem now stands the surgeon certainly has a hand in solving the problem and in the present unsatisfactory state of knowledge in him lies the most hopeful agent for relief.

The vast literature aimed at the solution of this problem has to do with experiments on animals, and on animals of unknown ages at that. Few experiments are positive beyond cavil, varying from animal to animal and differing much in the hands of different experimenters.

The paper by Boothby above cited contains 347 references, Wegelin's work (Schilddrüse, Band 8, Handbuch der Spec. Path., Anat. u. Hist., herausg. v. Henke-Lubarsch, Springer, Berlin, 1926) contains 540 pages and more references than one can count, almost all beyond the comprehension of a mere surgeon. Of comprehensive works of a practical nature Crotti's (Thyroid and Thymus, Lea and Febiger, Phila., ed. 2, 1922) and Joll's (Diseases of the Thyroid Gland, Mosby, St. Louis, 1932) works may be mentioned. After all the surgeon's best travelogue is a record of his journeys from the clinic to the laboratory multiplied by the number of days of his natural life.

Chapter IV

Nontoxic Diffuse Goiter
(Adolescent Goiter)

I N THE nontoxic diffuse goiters of early life we have the alphabet of all goitrous diseases. We have all its parts in its simplest forms. We have here not only the beginning as a physiologic disturbance but also the very earliest evidence of the changes that will later thrust themselves on our clinical attention in the various types of goiter.

We have in this form, seen only in early life, an enlargement that is due to a collection of colloid in the acini, nothing else. There is no cell proliferation and there being none the changes may be regarded as functional and capable of returning to normal. The accumulation of colloid is brought about by some disturbance of metabolism, lack of iodine or something of that sort. Though these changes antedate puberty, in many cases beginning before there is a general development of the other endocrine glands, they are most pronounced at that period of life. In the very beginning we find complications caused by the influence of other endocrine organs.

Though we accept as the prototype of nontoxic diffuse goiter, simple distention of the follicles with an excess of colloid, there are many variations which appear that must be noted. Various types of cell proliferation occur, not discernible in the clinic, which takes them out of the class of physiologic disturbances and places them in the pathologic class, for even in childhood they are started on the way of permanent mischief.

In children before puberty in most cases there is no cell proliferation and we have reason to assume the disturbance is only physiologic but there is a form, generally like the simple type, but which develops small papillary proliferations of epithelium which extend into the lumen of the distended acini without influencing the form of the goiter. That something is going on in the goiter is evidenced by the development of signs suggestive of exophthalmic goiter. They lack the general clinical and pathologic features of the disease in the adult consequently it seems proper to discuss them here since in general they resemble more the simple goiter of childhood than the Basedow of adults.

After a simple colloid goiter has existed for some time, due to unknown factors, small new follicles form in the walls of or between the old follicles.

The development of these is so insidious that the time of their beginning is not known. Since the form of the goiter is not notably influenced or the function not perceptibly disturbed these may remain in this simple group despite the fact that with the advent of such changes they are already entered into the first stage of nontoxic nodular goiters.

These variations make it desirable to discuss this group of goiters under three heads, the simple group described above; those in which there is papillation of the epithelium, consequently associated with eye changes; and those which are attended by the early signs of acinal proliferation.

These groups may be listed as follows:

    I. Colloid Goiter of Childhood Without Organic Change
   II. Colloid Goiters of Childhood with Papillary Formations
  III. Colloid Goiter with Acinal Proliferation

This list does not include the various developmental disturbances and degenerations which, though usually found in midlife, may also be found in childhood. These having a different clinical and pathologic import will be discussed in the chapter in which their characteristics align them, irrespective of age.

COLLOID GOITER OF CHILDHOOD WITHOUT
ORGANIC CHANGE

The calendar limits of childhood are a matter of perennial discussion in the great American home but acceptable conclusions are never reached. So it is with goiters. Childhood has no more definite limits in goiters than it has in social life. For purposes of discussion childhood must include the entire developmental period of life, rudely interrupted by puberty, to the final attainment of complete physical development.

The group of thyroid enlargements considered here fully justifies the title of this chapter, diffuse and nontoxic, being free from cell hyperplasia. These goiters being without cellular proliferation complete recovery is possible. Therefore if a goiter disappears and does not recur we know in retrospect that it was of this type. If it fails to disappear, or if having subsided it recurs, we know it contained areas of proliferation and will in time enter the nodular nontoxic stage. It is necessary therefore in the clinic to be constantly alert in anticipation of secondary changes lest our prognosis be too optimistic. We can only say in an abstract way, the younger the child the more likely is it to be simple. Before puberty it is likely to be free from evidence of proliferation but after that period of life it is progressively less likely to be simple until the full limit of adolescence, say at the twenty-eighth year, one may be certain that hyperplasia has begun.

Pathogenesis. What little we know about the genesis of goiter applies to this form. So far as our present purpose goes we may satisfy ourselves by conjecturing that some chemical disturbance causes colloid to accumulate in the acini. But the enigma of why, in the same environment, it accumulates in some thyroids and not in others shows how little we really know about what actually happens. Now since general inspection

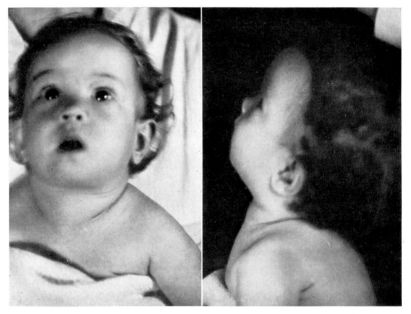

FIG. 49. Goiter in early life. It was uniform in size and consistency and disappeared spontaneously.

of school children has been instituted the surgeon is often consulted relative to the significance of a palpable thyroid. The first problem to be considered is whether there is an abnormal increase in the size of the gland. In slender children the normal thyroid is palpable. If firm to the touch one may assume that it is due to some physiologic change. In infants if the gland is visible it may be regarded as evidence of thyroid enlargement (Fig. 49).

Not all simple goiters are small. They may be of considerable size, say as large as a hen's egg, observed usually after puberty. Large goiters observed before puberty usually represent some developmental disturbance, hence most certainly do not belong to this group but are more or less related to the cretinoid state. That the larger ones, even when observed after puberty belong to this simple type one must say with reserve for failure to return to normal may invalidate our judgment. The

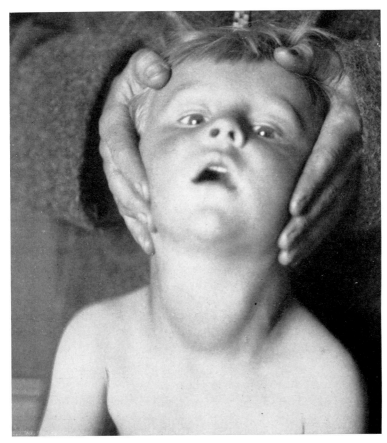

FIG. 50. The thyroid enlargement was apparently uniform but failed to disappear and later became nodular.

larger the goiters and the older the child the more likely it is that the goiter has developed areas of hyperplasia.

Even in children a goiter apparently uniform in the clinic (Fig. 50) may be nodular, due to degenerative changes. This possibility cannot be too strongly emphasized. Age of the child is no guarantee that the gland is uniform and of the simple type. In children fetal adenomas are easily enough felt as small isolated nodules.

The normal course of these simple colloid goiters is reversion to normal, often as puberty approaches, and with or without treatment. In other cases the thyroid enlargement is not manifest until the advent of puberty. In these cases the attempt at endocrine adjustment may cause enlargement of the thyroid gland. When this adjustment is achieved the goiter subsides. These patients present a uniform and somewhat firm thyroid enlargement. We may assume that the iodine content of the gland is insufficient to supply the need. In such cases there is often an associated dysmenorrhea.

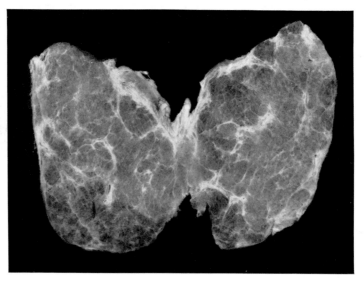

Fig. 51. Uniform colloid goiter in a child. The gland is uniform and the surface is imperfectly divided into areas by fibrous septa.

In other cases the thyroid gland is uniformly enlarged, distinctly soft to the touch and without other endocrine involvement. These also may disappear but the majority, though they may regress for a time, are prone to recur after a period of years. When this type subsides one never knows whether or not the recovery is permanent.

Pathology. Because these goiters are symptomless, material is not available by the operative route and only a chance autopsy provides material for anatomic study. After puberty the goiter not infrequently becomes so large that it is unsightly and the young people demand operative removal for cosmetic reasons.

On palpation these glands are uniform in outline and in consistency, a fact evident in the clinic and emphasized during the course of the operation. They are pale, almost translucent, and are readily separated from their environment.

On cross-section, the uniformity is maintained but the field is seen to be traversed by connective tissue septa dividing the area into more or less ovoid areas (Fig. 51) just as it is in normal glands. The translucency is emphasized and the larger acini may be apparent to the naked eye. A chance section may discover a fetal adenoma, but this is in no sense a part of the essential picture of a simple colloid goiter.

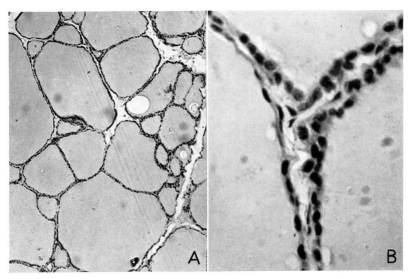

FIG. 52. Adolescent goiter, boy aged 14. *A*, General but unequal distention of the follicles. The colloid is uniform. *B*, The cells lining the acini are unequal, some normal, some flat and apparently functionless, and for small areas entirely absent.

Histology. The microscopic structure of these goiters is similar to that of the normal gland of persons of like age excepting that the acini contain more colloid than the normal. This accounts for the increase in the size of the gland, the increase corresponding exactly to the increase of the individual acini.

The acinal cells are uniform but flat and suggest a low state of activity (Fig. 52); and inasmuch as it is probable that such goiters can return to normal, these cells may be said to be in a resting state.

The colloid usually stains a paler pink than normal, though it is uniform in character. There may be a lack of tinctorial uniformity in the several acini, but a pronouncedly basic colloid is very rare in children.

A greatly varying degree of intensity of acid staining is occasionally observed. Deeply staining acini may lie beside the very faintly staining ones. That these represent different physiologic functions is evident, but what they are is not apparent.

A more detailed study of the acinal epithelium is worth while in view of what is to follow. The cells lining the acini, as above noted, are flat, the nuclei uniformly ovoid, the protoplasm more than normally sensitive to acid dyes. As in a normal gland, there are interspersed between the acini solid—or what appear to be solid—areas of cells lying between the

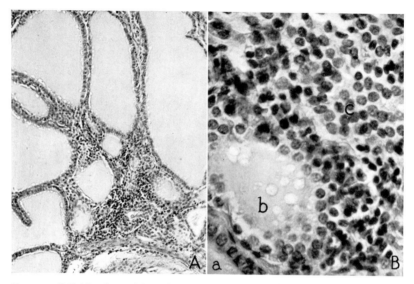

FIG. 53. Colloid goiter, girl aged 9. *A*, Acini unequally distended. The acinal cells are cuboid and uniform. *B*, Interacinal area of cells: *a*, normal acinus; *b*, illy formed acinus; *c*, mass of cells without lumina but which stain like those lining the acini.

acini (Fig. 53). The source of these and their purpose are matters of dispute; some writers even deny that one sees anything, ascribing it to an optical illusion.

COLLOID GOITER OF CHILDHOOD WITH PAPILLARY FORMATION

It was noted in the preceding section that simple nontoxic colloid goiters of adolescence were characterized by the entire absence of any cellular hyperplasia. In a few cases there are noted small knots of cellular hypertrophy which project into the lumina of the acini.

Children with goiters that apparently are like the simple colloid goiter, more or less suddenly without notable changes in the course, develop protrusion of the eyeballs. Until this complication occurs there is no notable difference. Though there is protrusion of the eyeballs, it would be a mistake to label these cases exophthalmic goiters, because the other symptoms which characterize that disease are lacking. There is entirely missing the stormy evidence of toxicity commonly seen in Graves' dis-

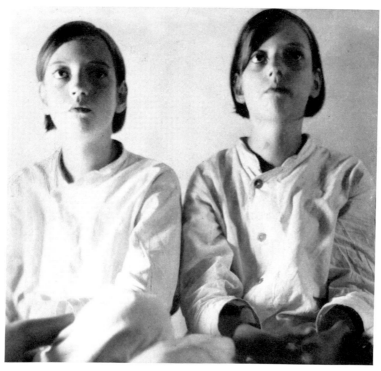

Fig. 54. Exophthalmos in twins. No goiter was visible but enlargement was evident on palpation. (Dr. Neff's patients.)

ease in adults. The eye signs begin so insidiously that not uncommonly this is the first sign that calls attention to the presence of a goiter. Usually, however, a simple goiter is recognized before the advent of the eye signs. Though the possibility of the appearance must be kept in mind in all cases, their occurrence is so rare that one is not justified in engendering apprehension in the parent by mentioning such a possibility. These goiters with eye signs occur in early life. My youngest patient was 2½ years old at the time of operation.

True Graves' disease does occur in childhood, but it is rare before puberty.

Pathogenesis. We have an abundance of theories as to the causation of exophthalmic goiter. We have none to explain the occurrence of exophthalmos in children. Perhaps this is an added reason for classifying them here, for here one can more easily assume that the cellular proliferation is due wholly to local causes.

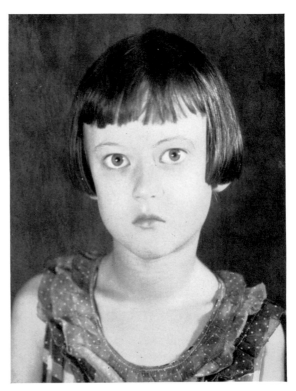

F IG. 55. Exophthalmic goiter in a child aged 5 years. The goiter is barely visible and the eye signs are not marked.

The eye signs may begin before the goiter is definitely palpable (Fig. 54), the associated nervousness may suggest chorea. Although there generally is an associated irritability and nervousness the patient may be tranquil and apparently undisturbed (Fig. 55). My experience is that these patients are unusually bright. Though there usually is an associated augmentation of pulse rate, there never is tremor nor vascular disturbance.

The usual eye sign is that of exophthalmos without the presence of other signs generally associated with exophthalmic goiter. It is this single feature of exophthalmos which concerns the surgeon. If neglected the protrusion of the eyeball may become permanent and assume such proportions that the conjunctiva is jeopardized. This all is hearsay—I have never seen a patient whose conjunctiva seemed to be endangered by the protrusion. I have, however, observed cases in which the increase of exophthalmos was so rapid that I feared to defer operation because of

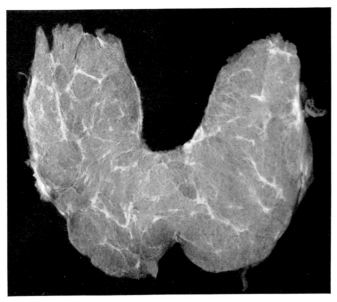

F IG. 56. Colloid goiter with exophthalmos in a boy aged 14. The gland has the appearance of simple colloid.

this possibility. Certain it is that the longer the exophthalmos is allowed to exist before operation the less likely it is to regress fully after operation. In this it follows the same law that prevails in the exophthalmic goiter of adults.

It has been my privilege to observe a number of these patients without treatment over several decades. Exophthalmos with moderately rapid pulse and perhaps with an increase of nervousness is all that is manifest. The natural apprehension of the mother sometimes seemed to be largely responsible for the increased nervousness. After many months the pulse slows and the exophthalmos remains stationary for a time; regresses to a certain degree and then remains stationary throughout life. In contrast, when an operation is performed the progression of the exophthalmos stops immediately and regresses inversely to its duration. One case observed for thirty years and then 'ectomized for interstitial goiter still showed the typical papillations of the infant exophthalmic goiter and there was some permanent protrusion of the eyeballs. Therefore, in the less pronounced cases the surgeon finds it difficult to decide which course to pursue. Regrets, in my experience, come most often from procrastination.

Whether there is a visible goiter or not, and even when there is no palpable gland, eye signs inform one that goiter is present and its extirpa-

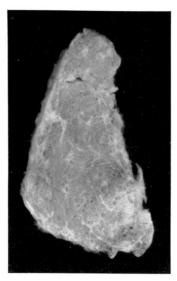

FIG. 57. Small colloid goiter more fibrous and redder than the preceding. Girl age 8.

tion may be necessary to relieve the exophthalmos. Nearly always, however, there is on palpation a goiter uniform in outline and in consistency.

Pathology. On palpation the gland does not differ from the simple colloid. When exposed at operation they are almost translucent and separate easily from their environment; there is no friability of tissue. There is nothing in the gross anatomy to distinguish them from the simple colloid goiters.

The cross-section of the gland does not differ from that of a simple colloid goiter (Fig. 56). The general color is pale, almost translucent; the larger the gland the more this is evident. If the gland is small it is usually firm and redder in color (Fig. 57). In rare cases multiple cysts are scattered throughout the gland. These are smooth walled and the contents light or straw colored, which hardens with the specimen. This condition exists only in those cases of a simple goiter which has existed a long time before the advent of the eye signs. The cysts are obviously only incidental.

Even though the general outline of the goiter be uniform even in this

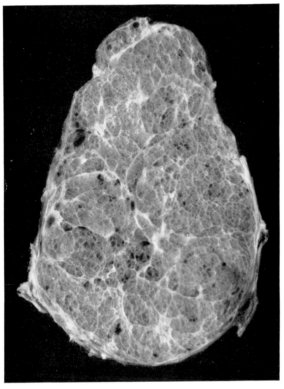

FIG. 58. Goiter with exophthalmos in a child aged 14. The surface of the section shows areas outlined by bundles of fibrous tissue, the general picture being that of ovoid areas.

early stage the cut surface shows division into fields by the fibrous septa which suggest the nodulations of later life (Fig. 58).

Histology. The microscopic examination makes clear the reason why these glands resemble so closely those of the simple goiters. For the most part the slides show the picture of a simple colloid goiter, enlarged acini and a low epithelium. The difference lies in the small areas in which there are papillary projections of epithelial cells into the lumen of the acini (Fig. 59). There is seldom any difficulty in distinguishing between

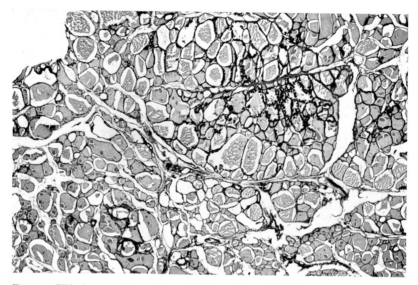

FIG. 59. Slide from a goiter with exophthalmos in a child of five. The majority of the acini are distended with uniform colloid. In a small area in the center small papillary projections extend into the acini. The greater part of the slide represents a simple colloid of childhood.

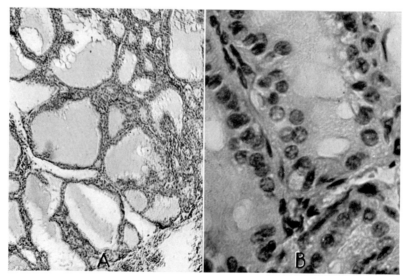

FIG. 60. Colloid goiter with exophthalmos. Slide from a small area showing hyperplasia: A, newly formed acini with beginning papillation; B, the same cells columnar, somewhat unequal. The colloid is palely staining and tends to vacuole formation.

these and the adult Graves' disease in the slide as there is none in the clinic. So small may be the area showing the papillations that they may be overlooked if a single block only is sectioned. If there are eye signs, there always are definite papillations somewhere.

Border-line cases are encountered, usually after puberty, which show early signs of true Graves' disease, tremor, vascular disturbance. These cases show evidence of new acinal formation (Fig. 60).

Small areas may sometimes be found that contain adenoid nodules about which are small acini with columnar epithelium. Such areas are

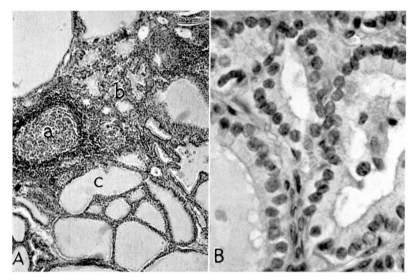

FIG. 61. Colloid goiter with eye signs, age 9, in a child with lymphoid nodules and newly formed acini: *A*, *a*, lymph nodule with germinal center, *b*, newly formed acini, *c*, colloid follicle moderately enlarged. *B*, Epithelium in the small acini. The cells are columnar and the nuclei are situated near the bases.

usually small and are generally overlooked unless diligently sought for. The presence of these nodules sometimes indicates unusually nervous states of the patient. Not uncommonly true lymph follicles are observed in these goiters (*A*, Fig. 61). These papillations are covered with cuboid or even columnar epithelium (*B*, Fig. 61) and there may be evidence of newly formed acini. Such cases are usually seen in older children, show greater nervous disturbance and may represent a tendency to the fully developed Graves' disease as seen in the adult.

COLLOID GOITER WITH ACINAL FORMATION

The reason for discussing this group apart from the simple colloid is that it either does not regress, or does so only imperfectly. The explanation for this is furnished by the slide. It reveals the formation of new acini, thus tending to the next stage, the nodular nontoxic.

They are without notable toxic symptoms, but the patients generally are nervous and irritable and few have a normal pulse rate. They are usually seen during the first few years after puberty but may extend to early adult life.

The distinctive characteristic of this group is hyperplasia, and once proliferation of acini begins there is no return to normal. There may be, it is true, a minor degree of regression, but not a recovery. I have had abundant opportunity to observe patients in their 'teens with simple goiter showing a diminution of their glands for a time, only to have them return and, after a period of symmetry, perhaps after repeated pregnancies, exhibit a bosselated goiter, simple or toxic.

That the gland is in a state of physiologic disturbance becomes probable when there is other evidence of endocrine imbalance, chiefly dysmenorrhea. In these when endocrine balance is achieved the size of the goiter lessens only to increase again at the time of gestation.

We have to do here with glands essentially simple colloid but with beginning cell proliferation. This point is useful to the operating surgeon for if, after a thyroidectomy, because of a large unsightly goiter, he finds in the slide these evidences of activity he may feel reasonably sure he has not seen the end of the trouble. Renewed or continued growth is spoken of as a recurrence. This may take the direction of a nodular nontoxic or a toxic goiter in subsequent years. Therefore the chief reason for insisting on the recognition of these newly formed acini is that it gives a better understanding of the consequence, notably the nontoxic colloid goiter.

That there is no dividing line between these and the bosselated colloids is, from the foregoing, self-evident. So long as they are smooth in outline to palpation and are uniformly elastic they belong to this group in the clinic. When they become bosselated or firm we know they have passed to the next group. The age of the patient is not a criterion though, of course, the younger the patient the less likely there is to be acinal proliferation. Conversely, the older the patient the more likely will the goiter be nodular in the laboratory, whatever may be the palpatory evidence in the clinic. It is impressive to remove the greater part of such a goiter—apparently a uniform goiter in the clinic—only to find it nodular on cross-section, and then have it return within a few years as a bosselated goiter.

Pathogenesis. It may be accepted that the cause of goiters is some disturbance in iodine metabolism but why they begin as simple distentions

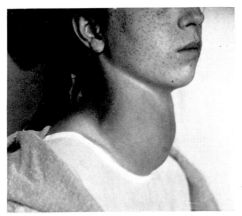

Fig. 62. Large colloid goiter in a girl of 15. First noticed five years before. Recurrence followed removal and became toxic seven years later after the patient had given birth to two children.

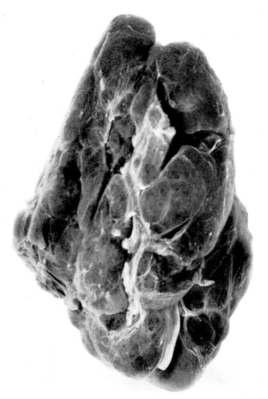

Fig. 63. Colloid goiter. Smooth in the clinic but nodular when removed.

of acini with colloid only to be followed by cell activity is a mystery but study of the histochemistry suggests the possibility that some alteration in the colloid permanently destroys the capacity of the epithelium to return to function and that the subsequent cellular changes are compensatory. The early appearance of basophilic colloid is the basis of this hypothesis.

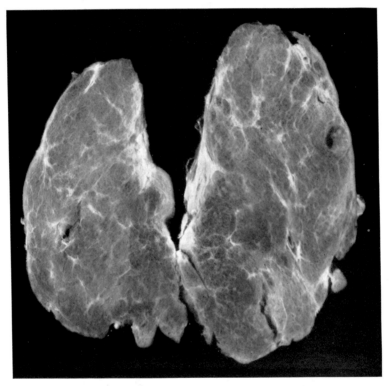

FIG. 64. Uniform colloid goiter from a girl aged 13. The surface is marked by the fibrous septa-like normal glands suggesting the first stage toward lobulations.

The large uniform goiters in young persons, in this region, comprise considerably less than one per cent of the total number of goiter cases observed. These few however present a rather striking picture. Observed over the years the soft goiters of early life continue to enlarge, still retaining their uniform outline and soft feel.

A large uniform goiter, soft and elastic throughout, without notable physical disturbance, is the picture of this stage of goiter. Though supposedly they present only a deformity without disturbing symptoms, the fact is that these patients are usually lacking in physical vigor and display the signs of irritability already mentioned.

The thyroid enlarges uniformly, producing a protruding mass quite apparent to the eye (Fig. 62). Generally it remains just that, an un-

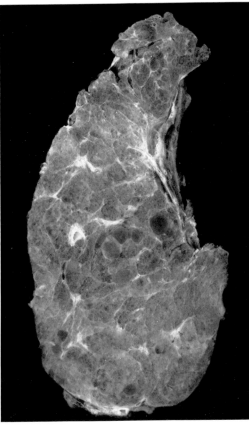

FIG. 65. Colloid goiter from a girl aged 16. The external surface is uniform but the gland is divided into round nodules lighter in color indicating a greater colloid content.

sightly mass which the patient resents, and which inspires her appeal to the surgeon. He must ask himself the question: If untreated what will the end be? Once the goiter becomes as large as that of the patient shown in the figure, any prospect of a spontaneous regression is very remote. If it remains stationary for a long period, particularly if it shows denser areas, there is little hope of spontaneous regression and none of complete recovery.

More slowly developing uniform colloid goiters are sometimes observed, particularly in men. These may exist for a period of years without notable change, retaining their simple structure. These may, rather unexpectedly, respond to medical treatment.

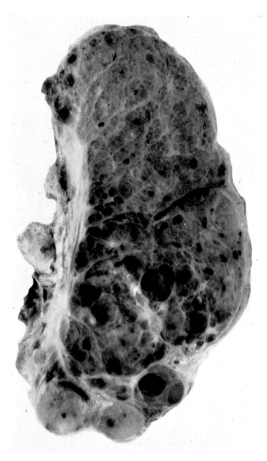

FIG. 66. Uniform colloid goiter in the clinic. The surface shows many incipient bosselations and below several which because of their situation escaped the examining fingers. Recurrence of Fig. 64.

It must be reiterated that the fact that a patient is in the adolescent age is no assurance that she has an adolescent, that is, a simple goiter. In this region of the country, the vast majority of goiters in adolescents are already bosselated on cross-section if not in the clinic. When this bosselation, evident only on cross-section, began there is no way of ascertaining.

The surgeon is confronted by a lesion in these goiters which is not going to regress but which is doing no notable mischief. His course will naturally be determined by what he believes to be the end stage.

Pathology. The simple goiter of early life in which hyperplasia has just begun is soft, almost semifluctuating to the touch, whether it be examined in the clinic or in the laboratory. It is pale pink, almost translucent. It gives the impression of a mass of colloid held together by thin plates and strands of connective tissue (Fig. 63). The reason is that it is just that.

In other cases even during the operation one perceives that the term "symmetrical" or "smooth" is a misnomer. The gland is neither. The

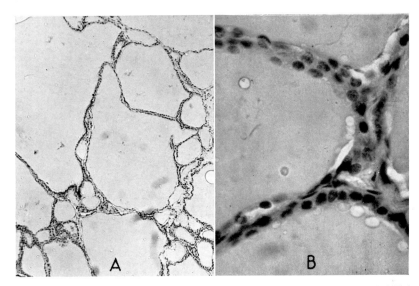

FIG. 67. Simple colloid goiter with the formation of new acini: *A*, the small follicles seem to be forming in the walls of the old follicles; *B*, the walls of the new follicles are lined by epithelium only slightly higher than that of the old follicles.

low bosselations already indicated in normal glands are emphasized in the goiter. It is well to fix this picture in one's eye, for it will aid in understanding the bosselations when they occur, since they represent a transition between the two groups.

Goiters showing the beginnings of acinal proliferation exhibit, on cut surface, a picture resembling simple colloids without proliferation (Fig. 64). Goiters apparently uniform to the touch, and even during operation, may show on cut surface an abundance of uniformly round nodules (Fig. 65) not yet large enough to influence the external surface or to qualify as nodular nontoxic goiter.

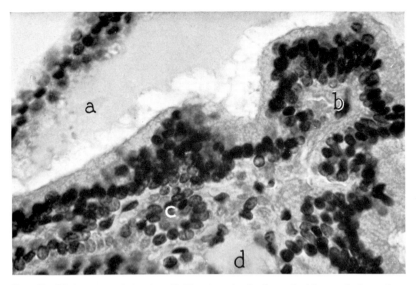

FIG. 68. High power of simple colloid goiter: beginning acinal hyperplasia; *a*, lumen of old acinus; *b*, pushing into the lumina of cells numerous and disarrayed; *c*, solid mass of cells in the interacinal area; *d*, attempt at acinus formation.

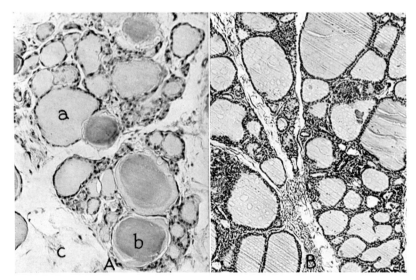

FIG. 69. Simple colloid goiter, girl, aged 16: *A, a*, the acinal epithelium is very flat; *b*, the contained colloid is basophilic; *c*, the fibrous tissue is prominent. *B*, The acinal epithelium is taller and masses of epithelium lie in the acinal interspaces.

Even on gross inspection the individual follicles surrounded by delicate partitions of connective tissue can be distinguished. The undulating outline of the capsule indicates the sites of future bosselation. From this capsule, bundles of connective tissue pass toward the center and mark off ever narrowing fields (Fig. 66).

Histology. The essential microscopic anatomy of these goiters is that of the simple colloid goiters, follicles distended with colloid, but there are in addition interspersed newly formed follicles at the border of the old (Fig. 67).

How these new acini form in the walls of the old becomes apparent on higher power. There seems to be a piling up of the epithelium of the old acini (Fig. 68). Other areas seem to be forming new acini from cells, probably interacinal cells left over from the developmental period. Be this as it may, this is the picture of the earliest deviation of the cell arrangement which ultimately ends in the various nodulations.

Even in very young persons some areas show changes transcending those corresponding to their years. The epithelium is exceedingly flat and the colloid discloses variations in stainability and may be distinctly basophilic (Fig. 69). Usually fibrosis may be added. Some of these have collections of cells in the interacinal spaces.

Literature

Goiter in Children. The surgical pathology of goiter in children finds but little expression in literature because they are so seldom subjected to operation. Exophthalmic goiters in children are now generally operated on. Although the pathology is not particularly emphasized a number of papers representing this phase may be quoted: McGraw (*Surg., Gynec. and Obst.*, July 1928, 47, 25–31), Green and Mora (*Ibid.*, Sept. 1931, 53, 375–77), Curtis (*Surg. Clin. N. Am.*, Feb. 1932, 12, 197–203), Abbott (*Internat. Clinics*, 1932, 42, 99–109), Rankin and Priestley (*West. J. Surg.*, Sept. 1932, 40, 498–505), Dinsmore (*J. A. M. A.*, Aug. 20, 1932, 99, 636–8) and Jackson (*Journal-Lancet*, Dec. 1933, 53, 635-639).

CHAPTER V

Nontoxic Nodular Goiter

(*Bosselated Goiter, Nontoxic Adenoma of Plummer*)

THE nodular nontoxic goiters may be defined as that group which forms nodules grossly recognizable, but without toxic signs that are apparent to the examiner. It is therefore purely a clinical term which has in mind only one factor of thyroid disease, namely toxicity. It does not take into consideration the fact that a goiter may cause injury to the patient without there having been at any time evidence of hyperthyroidism. It ignores wholly the histologic changes which they undergo.

In the broader sense because of the anatomic changes there is some question as to whether there is any such a thing as a nontoxic nodular goiter. If it is nodular it is hyperplastic, of that there is no doubt, and if it is hyperplastic it most certainly is toxic in the sense that it is injuring the patient, whether this be clinically manifest or not.

Yet the term is useful in the clinic. It covers in an indefinite way the span between the adolescent goiter on one hand and the more easily recognizable toxic state of the nodular toxic on the other. It is clinically significant in a broad way because the nodulations formed, restoration to normal is no longer possible. However the age of the patient is more important in the diagnosis than the detection in the clinic of bosselations because after the adult age is reached the characteristic changes have taken place whether the goiter has become nodular or not. In using the term therefore it should be kept in mind that it represents a stage of the disease and external form is not a characteristic feature. This is obvious in those cases which are uniform externally yet show nodules on cross-section.

Though a number of terms have been applied to this group, the term "nontoxic nodular" adopted by the Nomenclature Committee of the American Society for the Study of Goiter, may be accepted as the least objectionable of those proposed. This chapter discusses only the phase which has to do with the question of thyrotoxicity. The changes which find expression in constitutional disturbances will be discussed in a subsequent chapter (VII) but frequent references to them here cannot be avoided.

In the preceding chapter it was noted that in many, particularly in the older adolescents, there was already a tendency to form new acini. The same process is more pronounced here and it comes to dominate the picture for it is an extension of this process which leads to the formation of the nodules which are supposed to dominate the type of goiter now under consideration. The chief difficulty, from the pathologic viewpoint, arises when we attempt to determine whether the nodules are hyperplasias or adenomas. The nodules were heretofore called adenomas and it is the chief merit of the new nomenclature that this term is now avoided. The chief objection to the use of the term "adenoma" lies in the fact that it resulted in the quite general confusion of this type of nodule with the fetal adenomas, which are congenital. If that term must be used the chief objection could be eliminated by calling them secondary adenomas, in contradistinction to the congenital tumors which might then be called primary adenomas.

Be this as it may the nontoxic nodular goiter represents a midstage between the diffuse nontoxic colloid goiters of childhood and adolescence and the toxic colloid of midlife. The reason for discussing them as a special group lies in the fact that, in antithesis to the adolescent goiters, they are characterized by a dominant progressive tissue hyperplasia. Anatomically, therefore the nontoxic nodular goiter shows its beginning in the early histologic changes, before there is any clinical evidence of nodule formation. The stage ends when the degree of toxicity attains a stage where its presence cannot be doubted. The change from the nontoxic to the toxic is one of degree rather than of kind, so gradual is the change.

The nontoxic nodular goiter used as a clinical term, is dependent on the presence of bosselations perceptible to the examiner in the clinic and on the absence of signs of toxicity so far as the particular examiner can perceive. Obviously nodules large enough to be grossly discernible represent an advanced stage of the changes which cause the formation of the nodules. It would be simpler from the pathologic point of view to think of these goiters as diffuse colloid goiters of the adult in which sooner or later nodules will form for the age of the patient is more constant than the external form of the goiter. When a colloid goiter is found in the adult one may be sure that the fundamental processes which characterize this group are present and there is no need to emphasize the nodulosity or the absence of toxicity as a group characteristic.

The term "toxic" is universally used as a synonym of hyperthyroidism meaning that the goiter is hyperactive. That a goiter may be toxic because of degenerative changes which are taking place in it in the absence of cellular hyperplasia is obvious. It is necessary to keep this in mind. otherwise there is difficulty in explaining the signs from a study of the slide. It cannot be too strongly emphasized that the goiter may injure the patient without there being evidence of hyperthyroidism in the ordinary sense. The toxicity of degeneration may be active without the presence of hypersecretion.

Toxicity in the sense of a hypersecretion or of degeneration obviously begins before it is clinically recognized as such. Just how toxic must a nontoxic goiter become before it is toxic to the clinician? If one antici- pates the development of a clinical sign it will be recognized earlier than if one is oblivious of its ultimate advent. One may be sure that such a goiter will become toxic sooner or later.

If one studies the early nodular colloid goiters as one sees them in the clinical examination of patients, one thing stands out plainly: they are not free from disturbances of some kind. Usually the pulse rate is in- creased from 80 to 90 in persons who deny any disturbance from the goiter. A normal pulse rate in a person with a nodular goiter is a rarity even though it be clinically classed as nontoxic. This is nearly always accompanied by some nervous instability or irritability. It is necessary to accept these two factors together with the enlarged thyroid as the common accompaniment of the nontoxic nodular goiter. That is, the nontoxic goiter is already slightly toxic but not to a degree sufficient to impress either the patient or the doctor, except when one or the other or both are looking for some toxic manifestations. That these subdued dis- turbances are due to a beginning increased cellular activity is made evident by the structural change in the gland and by the fact that the complaints cease after the goiter is removed.

In rare instances, it is true, one finds nodular goiters that present none of the early signs of toxicity just mentioned. This type is prone to form soft pendulous goiters which are inconvenient only because of their size. These goiters are usually cystic, at least in part.

If one has the opportunity of observing such patients at intervals for a decade or two, he observes variations in the clinical picture. The early signs of toxicity, increased pulse rate and slight nervousness, may con- tinue with variations for many years. A series of exacerbations and re- missions is commonly observed before the patient becomes seriously enough incapacitated to warrant classification as toxic in ordinary clinical examination. The advent of toxicity should be recognized before it be- comes incapacitating.

It is worth noting that a nontoxic goiter is classed as toxic by both patient and doctor much earlier now than was the case even ten years ago. It is my conviction that in another decade the attempt to distinguish between the nontoxic and the toxic will be entirely abandoned. There is no anatomical warrant for such a separation into two groups and the experienced clinician ignores it. This is most emphatically the case when the surgeon combines his clinical observation with study in the laboratory. For him there is no nontoxic goiter beyond, say, the twenty-fifth year.

The whole problem of relative toxicity has been confused by an undue dependence on the basal rate. It would be fine if we could say that the toxic state is reached when the basal metabolic rate is elevated. At best the basal rate is elevated only in thyrotoxic cases due to cellular hyperplasia attended by increased metabolism. The basal rate does not measure the toxicity of degeneration and gives no warning of the progress toward a damaged heart.

The essential thing is to detect impending toxicity before there is heart damage. It is desirable to do this before the disease has advanced to a stage when the signs are pathognomonic of a toxic state. Early recognition of a stage tending to a serious lesion is as important in goiters as it is in the case of malignant tumors.

The anatomic study of this group is concerned with the genesis of toxicity rather than with the bosselations themselves. These are, as above noted, not always perceptible and are wholly unessential concommitants but once they are recognizable we may know that the cellular hyperplasia is well advanced.

We may start with the simple and uniform colloid of childhood and postulate a "resting" epithelium. If it rests too long the colloid commences to change and then hyperplasia begins. We need not expect, and we do not find, a great structural difference between the nontoxic colloid goiter and the later stages of the simple colloid goiter of adolescence in terms of active epithelium. There is some new formation of acini but no notable change in the cell form. We do not find the cellular changes which attend hypersecretion. In the search for changes in structure we must search elsewhere, notably in the colloid, for explanation of the signs observed in the clinic. It should be remembered also that the goiter is aging as is the patient and that the natural changes incident to advancing years are to be expected in both. It is difficult to decide sometimes which changes are due to development of the goiter and which are simply due to advancing years of the patient.

In summary one may say that the nontoxic nodular goiters do not represent a stage of innocence but the threshold of more important changes which will surely come in the advancing years. Instead of presenting a state that may be complacently ignored it represents a time when we can most surely rid the patient permanently of a serious malady.

Pathogenesis. In this chapter in order to keep in line with the generally accepted nomenclature we must regard nodular nontoxic goiters as those which on palpation present surfaces which are irregular. As indicated in a preceding chapter the nontoxic nodular goiters are closely associated with the nontoxic diffuse type—or stage, if you prefer. The most reliable clinical guide however to this type is not the nodulations but the age of the patient. In patients, say, of 25 or more years of age, the stage of the nontoxic nodular, pathologically considered, has been reached, regardless of whether or not the goiter can be perceived to be nodular. If it is not nodular in the clinic it will be when cut across in the laboratory. There are exceptions, of course, but nevertheless this is the most reliable guide we have at present. Most clinicians recognize the fact that when this age is reached there is no regression to normal because hyperplasia has begun and this is the criterion of advance to the next developmental stage which may antedate by a long period the formation of clinically recognizable nodulations. Certainly there is no need to delay the diagnosis until bosselations are perceptible in the clinic.

The converse is not true for patients under the age above mentioned are by no means always in the nonhyperplastic stage. It is not uncommon to find, even in the early adolescent period, glands of a type usually not present until midlife. These glands, it may be said, have passed prematurely to a hyperplastic stage.

Why goiters go on to this stage we are wholly without knowledge. All that is possible to do is to trace in an imperfect way how it comes about. This is possible only insofar as we can determine it by examining the various stages as operations supply the material and piecing the pictures together. Obviously we cannot follow the same case, except in rare cases when repeated operations are done.

Harking back to the days when goiter was a medical disease, I recall the following pictures. An adolescent patient presented herself possessed of a goiter. In many cases the goiter was discovered incidentally while examining the patient for other complaints. The goiter was regarded as innocent, of course. The goiter may have continued unchanged or it may have regressed, possibly disappeared. Five or ten years later the goiter, still innocent of course, had become generally irregular in outline sometimes nodulated. With an increasing number of pregnancies the bosselations grew in size and number. Many of these patients experienced periods of indisposition, sometimes requiring periods of rest. They may have had a nervous breakdown. Partial or apparently complete recovery

followed only perhaps to experience a relapse. Finally even despite varying degrees of weight loss, nervousness and pounding of the heart the
toxicity of the goiter was not recognized and we signed them out as dead
from cardiac disease, and we were far more nearly right than we suspected. The patients did die of heart disease, but we did not recognize
that the goiter was the cause of the failing heart.

Looking over records of 30 or 40 years ago I discover that a normal
pulse rate in patients in the nontoxic stage was a rare thing. I am convinced that anyone who will look over his records of equal antiquity
will become convinced that if evidence had been collected first and the
conclusions arrived at afterwards we might have avoided the error of
believing that there is a really nontoxic stage.

One reason we failed, and still fail, to recognize the early toxic signs
is that we have only the toxicity of hypersecretion in mind, failing even
now to recognize the toxicity of degeneration.

Just why goiters once established pursue an unremitting course to
the same end transcends our understanding. There is no other disease
which displays such an unrelenting regularity for so many years. Only
by comparing the advancing goiter with the degenerative changes in the
thyroids of normal persons do we get a lead.

Though ignorant of the causes operative in producing the disease,
there is one phase about which the surgeon can speak with confidence.
The nontoxic goiter will become toxic, toxic enough in fact to please
everybody and after a period of years it will menace the patient so seriously that operative removal will be urgently indicated, because of the
so anxiously anticipated toxicity. Here again the calendar has, in the
past, served a useful purpose. It has been estimated that in general a
nontoxic goiter becomes sufficiently toxic in about 16 years to necessitate
removal.

We have to do here, therefore, with a goiter which is nodular and
nontoxic only in a hyperthyroid sense. There is a constantly advancing
toxicity of degeneration which is even more fatal than the toxicity of
hypersecretion.

The subjective change which accompanied the toxicity of degeneration
is an indefinite nervousness often referred to as an "inward nervousness."
It manifests itself in irritability over things which previously passed
unnoticed. The severe forms of nervousness are referred to as "nervous
breakdowns," meaning thereby a nervousness which incapacitates the
patient. These nervous states are unlike the nervousness of hypersecretion which present unmistakable objective signs.

The early nervous symptoms are recognizable by the surgeon only by what the patient tells him about herself. Recognition of these more or less obscure symptoms is much facilitated if, given a goiter in an adult, such symptoms are sought for. The importance of suspecting this type of goiter lies in the fact that the subjective symptoms are not impressive and are likely to continue much the same mild course for many years. This leaves an interval during which conservative treatment may be justified when there are certain contraindications to operation, such as

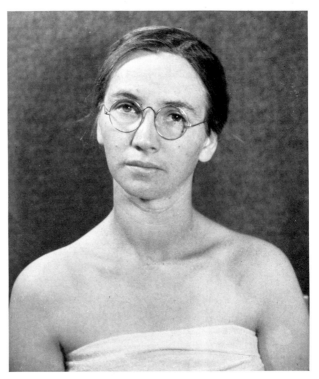

FIG. 70. Nodular nontoxic goiter. Matron, age 31. The enlargement surrounds the trachea in a uniform manner.

nursing a child, an impending high school commencement, or any of other numerous ordinary complications incident to normal family life. This indefinite and variable state is what we really mean by a nontoxic goiter. The toxicity has not yet reached a stage when, from our present viewpoint, we can say it demands operation without delay.

On the other hand hyperplasia of the acini may supervene and we have added to the mild toxicity of degeneration that of hypersecretion associated with the usual signs of an acutely toxic goiter.

If we attempt to translate these general statements into the experience of the clinic we meet a variable picture. The patient may present a pronounced uniform enlargement of the neck (Fig. 70). It encircles the trachea uniformly. This uniform enlargement naturally is more commonly observed in early adult life, for then the bosselations have not yet reached a clinically recognizable size because it takes time to produce

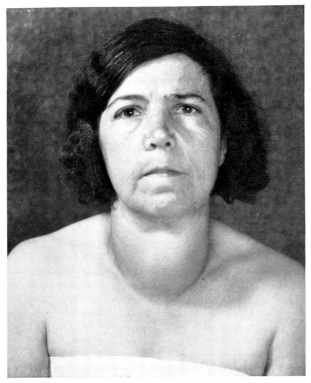

FIG. 71. Nodular nontoxic goiter. Matron, age 45. Protrusions appear on either side of the neck and at the isthmus.

a nodule of sufficient dimensions to convince those who believe a nodule is an essential feature. Later in life there becomes apparent an unevenness of surface due to large indefinite fullness in the several regions of the neck (Fig. 71). When a distinctly rounded nodule is apparent it generally is a fetal adenoma which may more or less obscure a nodulated enlargement of both lobes lying in the neck (Fig. 72).

In extreme cases the nodulations may be so large that they are actually pendent (Fig. 73). These cases are likely to be the least toxic of all, for these huge nodules are largely cystic and consequently lack parenchymatous tissue.

The external form as seen in the clinic has little to do with determining the type of goiter. The characteristic feature is a goiter usually of some size, firm but not hard, movable under the overlying muscles, and without notable sensitiveness to pressure. It is in truth an old colloid

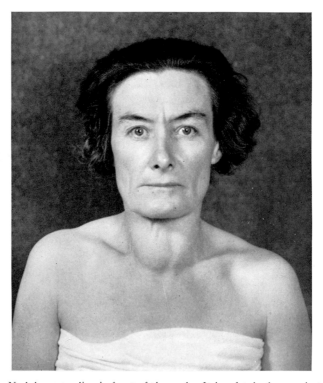

FIG. 72. Nodule protruding in front of the neck. It is a fetal adenoma but there was enlargement of each lobe the size of a hen's egg.

goiter of some years' duration, regardless of what the surface may reveal on inspection. This has very little reference to what the cross-section will show.

Physical changes associated with degenerations within the goiter may result in hemorrhage causing a sudden enlargement and tenderness, but do not necessarily portend increased toxicity. These are accidental changes unrelated to the problem of toxicity, but they do serve the useful purpose of sending the patient in a receptive mood to the surgeon.

So far as toxicity goes, the transition into the definitely toxic stage is usually slow, months and often years elapsing ere the change becomes impressive. On the other hand, acutely toxic stages may develop rapidly and, in rare hyperacute cases, death occurs within several weeks though there have been no warning signs of increasing toxicity. Because of the possibility of such a sudden onslaught of severe toxicity, the innocence of the slightly nontoxic stage should not be regarded with too great equanimity. I was once asked by a dying patient, the victim of a hyper-

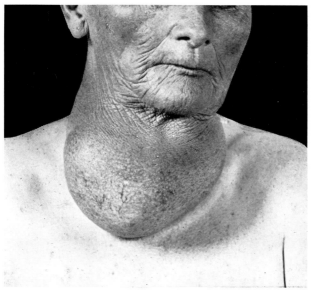

FIG. 73. Nodular nontoxic goiter. The lobes on the right side were so large that they were actually pendent.

acute attack, why she had not been operated on before the serious stage developed. I have been working on the answer for more than twenty years.

A nodular nontoxic goiter, in the sense here considered, is clinically one somewhere between the adolescent goiter and that of toxicity. Whatever the state at the time of observation we know with certainty that a menacing toxicity will be reached in the course of time. When this time comes the signs will be expressive of indefinite general symptoms, signs of hyperthyroidism of a more or less classical type, or the gradually developing cardiac decompensation. Whatever the route a particular goiter may take the end will be death from heart failure. That is the normal end of all goiters.

Pathology. The study of the pathology must of course begin with the palpation of the goiter while it still is *in situ*. The elastic feel and the smooth gliding surface are characteristic of nontoxic nodular goiter. All the lobules and the various parts of the goiter have a similar con-

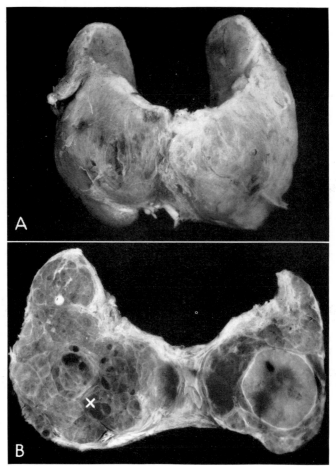

Fig. 74. Early nodular nontoxic goiter, age 38. *A*, The outline of the gland is uniform. *B*, On cross-section there are distinct bosselations. At *x*, is a fetal adenoma.

sistency. Since the softness of the uniform nontoxic continues through the nodular nontoxic and finally disappears with advancing toxicity of the toxic nodular, the degree of firmness is in a measure the gauge as to how near the nontoxic has approached the nodular toxic. The character of this feel is so distinctive that its importance cannot be overestimated.

It is worth more than a whole factory full of basal metabolic machines.

When the gland is exposed at operation the physical findings above detailed are verified. The goiter is easily separated from its environment unless it is fixed by lobules that have insinuated themselves between adjacent muscles or into the thoracic cavity.

Their relatively innocuous character is further manifest by the comparatively slight dilatation of the blood vessels, the firmness of the capsule and by the color of the gland.

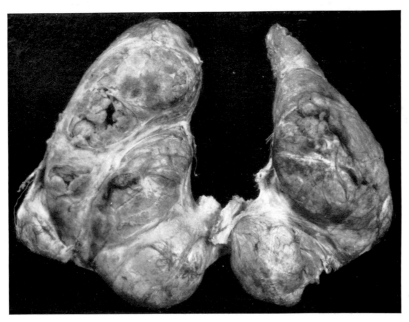

FIG. 75. Nodular nontoxic colloid goiter. The bosselations are low, barely to be made out as such in the clinic.

The early stages of the nodular toxic deviates very little from the uniform nontoxic (Fig. 74). The typical nodular goiter, the earliest recognizable in the clinic, is one whose surface presents numerous low bosselations (Fig. 75), which give little intimation as to the structure within the capsule. In more pronounced cases the nodules are so large they feel like a bag of potatoes (Fig. 76). It need scarcely be noted that size has nothing to do with the approach toward toxicity. In fact the contrary is true. These huge nodules, as already mentioned, are made up of degenerated or cystic cavities and consequently may show little tendency to become progressively toxic. Goiters in very old persons are usually of this type; the explanation being that they have not already died from a more rapidly progressive type.

The real study of the pathology begins with the cross-section. The greatest variety of gross pictures are encountered.

The least degree of changes presents a picture closely resembling the adolescent colloids (Fig. 77). There is little or no indication of the for-

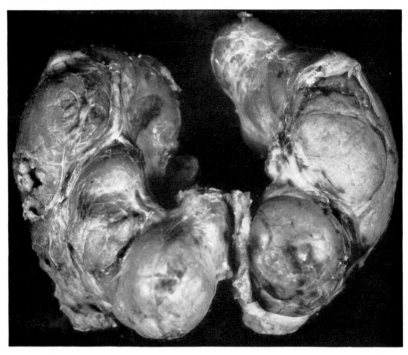

FIG. 76. Nodular nontoxic goiter. The nodules are large and were evident to the naked eye and to palpation.

mation of bosselations, the field being divided only by the fibrous septa. The general architecture is quite similar to that of the adolescent colloids in that large acini are recognizable with the naked eye, indicating that the hyperplasia is very little advanced. A goiter of corresponding external form may show an entirely different architecture. Although the nodulations may be small they are definitely outlined, there is a more advanced fibrosis and the whole surface is darker in color (Fig. 78). Individual acini can no longer be made out because of the more advanced hyperplasia. Not uncommonly this type advances to the nodular toxic stage without change in form. Such goiters are firmer because the connective tissue is more abundant and degenerative changes more advanced.

On the other hand, the surface may be pronouncedly nodular, the color reddish pink, more or less translucent as in adolescent colloid goiters, and some areas may show individual follicles so large that they can be discerned with the naked eye (Fig. 79). This type is prone to attain a large size and may show no evidence of toxicity for many years. These most completely fit the designation "nontoxic."

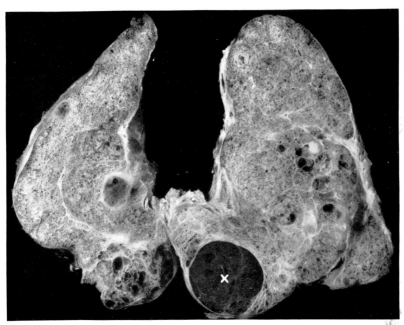

FIG. 77. Nontoxic nodular goiter. The nodulations are but little indicated but the white area indicates activity. At *x* is a fetal adenoma in an advanced stage of degeneration.

In most cases as the gland becomes older the fibrous septa increase in thickness, making apparent beginning bosselations. In these, individual acini are very large and may attain the size of veritable cysts. Often the several parts of the gland show structural variations, one part being nodular, the other part diffuse. The non-nodular areas usually show a nearer approach to toxicity than the nodular portions (Fig. 80).

Not infrequently distinct fetal adenomas are imbedded in the colloid as shown in several of the figures. These are congenital and they can be differentiated from the nodular by their developing as a part of a colloid goiter, though they may ultimately converge, when distinction may depend on microscopic study.

Histology. In studying the microscopic appearance of the nodular nontoxic goiters, we may hark back to the preceding chapter and note that there are new acini formed about the borders and between the acini. With the advent of the nodular form we have to deal with an exaggeration of that same process. As the toxic nodular stage is approached the evidence of hyperplasia increases.

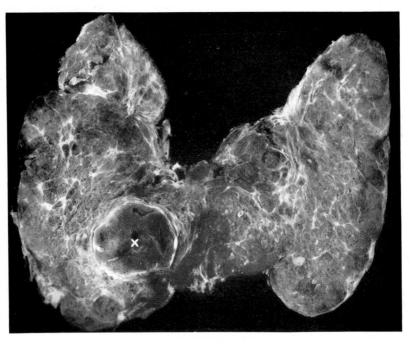

FIG. 78. Old colloid with a fairly uniform surface. The cut surface is divided into many minute nodules by prominent connective tissue septa. At x is a fetal adenoma.

We may pause here to study how the nodulations develop. This has already been briefly referred to in the chapter on general pathology. We saw there that the first step toward nodulations is the formation of new acini in the wall of the old ones or in the spaces between several acini. Not only do new acini develop but the old acini become so hugely dilated as to almost attain cystic dimensions (Fig. 81). These larger acini, or cysts, are not spheroidal, indicating that their contents are not under any considerable pressure. As nodules form some are compressed when adjacent nodules display greater activity, indicated by the abundant new acinal formation, the new spheroidal form and greater stainability of the cells (Fig. 82). The new nodules may be made up of many small acini, hence these areas may imitate the fetal adenomas (Fig. 83).

The progress of the nontoxic goiter is marked by the increasing changes in the colloid. The changes may be so great that it stains blue with hematoxylin. Lesser changes stain more or less with eosin but with Mallory's aniline blue the colloid stains an orange color instead of blue as in the normal colloid (Fig. 84).

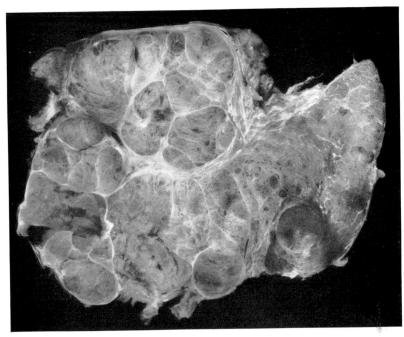

FIG. 79. Nontoxic nodular goiter. The nodules are defined by distinct septa. The large pale nodules bespeak nontoxicity. Large cystic areas can be made out.

One may say in a general way also that the microscopic differences between the nontoxic nodular goiter and the nodular toxic is shown in the greater activity of the acinal cells. There are, in addition to new acini of the nontoxic state, acini lined with cells of much greater activity. As this stage approaches the toxic the evidence of cellular activity becomes more and more impressive. Quite commonly, as the stage of bosselation is reached, the greater part continues to present the picture of the nontoxic (*A*, Fig. 85). Here and there are found islands of acini showing more deeply staining cells (*B*, Fig. 85). While areas of cells are found which are larger and stain more deeply than the cells in the early colloid state they lack the uniform enlargement and stainability of the hyperplastic hyperthyroid state. As toxicity nears the same picture

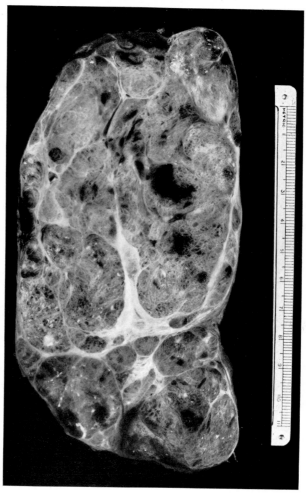

FIG. 80. Old colloid goiter divided by heavy fibrous tissue septa. Many of the acini are visible to the naked eye.

becomes more noticeable (Fig. 86). While the cells are larger and stain more deeply they are irregular in size and stainability and suggest more the cellular arrangement of a neoplastic growth than they do the hyperplasia of a thyrotoxic goiter. Sometimes small areas show a regular

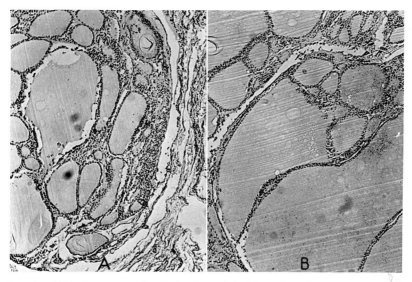

FIG. 81. Slide from an early distinctly nodular nontoxic goiter: *A*, the acini are moderately enlarged and there are many newly formed acini about the periphery. At the border old acini are compressed to form a pseudocapsule for the nodule; *B*, several of the acini have attained huge proportions.

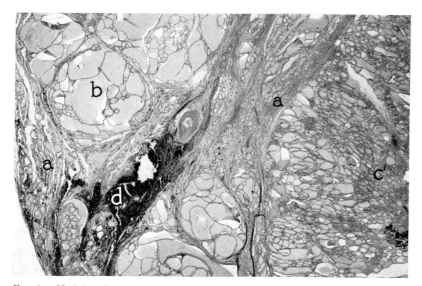

FIG. 82. Nodulated nontoxic goiter: *a,a*, area of compressed acini; *b*, very large acini; *c*, more active nodule as indicated by the more numerous small acini and the greater stainability of the cells; *d*, area in which the structure is obscured by hemorrhage.

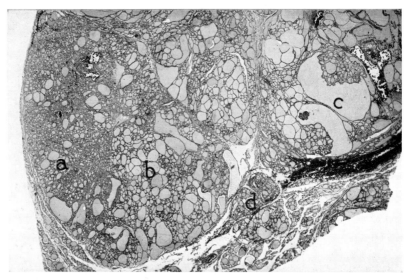

FIG. 83. Newly developed acini in a nodular nontoxic goiter: *a*, area made up of very small acini; *b*, acini of normal size and spheroidal; *c*, a large acinus with a multitude of small acini protruding into its lumen; *d*, areas compressed to form a capsule.

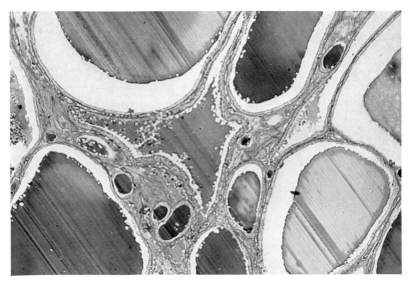

FIG. 84. Nontoxic nodular goiter. Female, age 29. Early changes of degenerative toxicity. The epithelium is little changed. The colloid stained normally with eosin but with aniline blue the colloid shows various changes in tinctorial reaction and there is a tendency of retraction.

arrangement of cells in some acini but the cells stain more deeply than in the hyperplasia of thyroid hyperactivity. Such changes are always associated with degenerated colloid.

Some authors have seized on these acini as evidence that they are the source of the formation of the nodules (Fig. 87) and on this theory have called the nodules adenomas. This cannot be, because the nodules are formed long before such fields are seen. These areas are seen only as the goiter is definitely approaching the toxic stage. They are particularly likely to be found in patients who have a toxic spell and then emerge

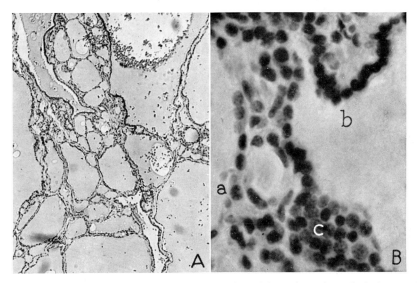

FIG. 85. Early approach to toxicity in nontoxic nodular goiter: *A*, typical picture of early stage; *B*, areas of more deeply staining cells, *a*, acinus with flat cells; *b*, acinus with taller more deeply staining cells; *c*, masses of cells without a lumen.

into a more quiescent stage. Certain it is that areas showing such active cells are not found during the years of nontoxicity and they do not form the nodulations. Just why some areas develop nodules while other areas are compressed serving to form capsules for the more active areas is not known. But this confession of ignorance is at least one step nearer the truth than theories which force adenoma formation from structures that do not exist.

Becoming toxic is not the most mischievous change these goiters undergo. Instead of indulging in increased cellular activity with ensuing toxicity production, they degenerate, and the patient passes directly into the cardiotoxic state.

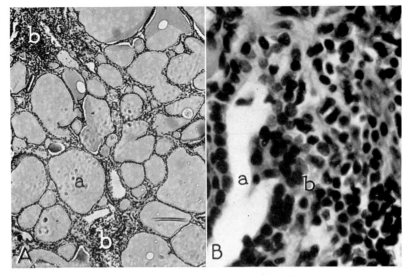

FIG. 86. Advanced nontoxic nodular goiter: *A,a,* acinus lined with flat epithelium; *b,b,* nodules of more deeply staining cells; *B,* high power of same, *a,* an acinus with cuboidal deeply staining cells with indifferent colloid; *b,* masses of deeply staining cells and a few with pale ovoid nuclei.

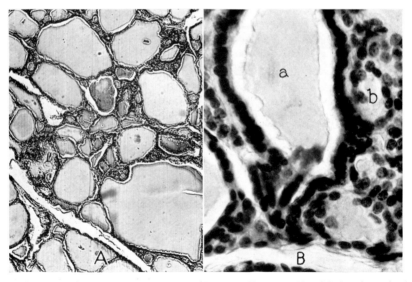

FIG. 87. Nontoxic nodular stage: *A,* acini with fibrous walls with low imperfectly staining cells. Between these are more active areas; *B, a,* acinus with columnar deeply staining epithelium; *b,b,* small space containing colloid, surrounded by less deeply staining cells.

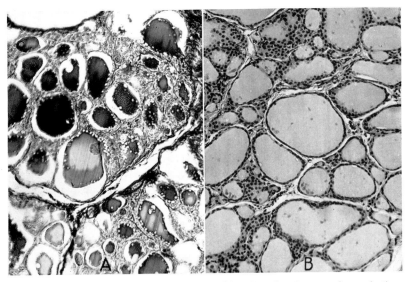

FIG. 88. Degenerating colloid goiter: *A*, colloid undergoing degeneration as indicated by the tinctorial changes in the colloid, the very flat acinal epithelium; *B*, small acini, the colloid of which is uniformly staining. There are many cells lying between the acini.

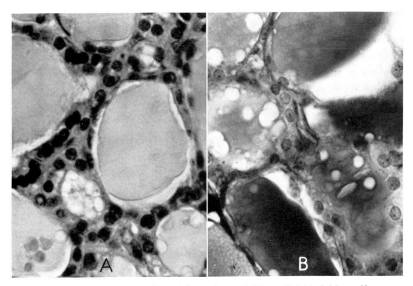

FIG. 89. Degenerating nontoxic nodular goiter. *A*, The colloid is fairly uniform; some acini lined by deeply staining cells, others degenerated or absent. *B*, The colloid is in an advanced state of degeneration, the acinal cells degenerating or entirely absent.

The first indications of degeneration are changes in the tinctorial reaction of the colloid. Some are more densely staining, some mottled, some scarcely stainable at all (*A*, Fig. 88), some intensely basophilic. Such areas may embrace very small space at first, the greater part of the goiter being made up of ordinary colloid goiter (*B*, Fig. 88). Gradually, however, more and more of the total area becomes involved. These are the changes of a cardiotoxic goiter and not of thyrotoxicity. One may find combinations of activity and degeneration of cellular activity (*A*, Fig. 89) and other areas showing an advanced stage of degeneration (*B*, Fig. 89).

Unsatisfactory as may be our knowledge of the histopathology of this stage of goiter, a careful study of the gland in the laboratory is a more accurate guide in appraising the patient's state than is the clinical. When areas are found like those shown in the last figure one may be surprised by cardiac arrhythmias which were not in evidence before the operation. This is likely to be the case in long standing cases in old matrons who deny any complaint but some still small voice tells them that it is time to seek relief.

Literature

Nontoxic Nodular Goiter. How the nodulations form has always been a puzzle. Aschoff (Lectures on Pathology, Hoever, New York, 1924) discusses their development but I have never been able to grasp his meaning. The central canaliculi which he has assumed to form the basis I have seen only twice in many thousand nodular goiters. On this basis he declares the nodules as true tumors. If so they present characteristics not possessed by any other tumors, benign or malignant, namely they invariably undergo degeneration in a specific progressive way. Hellwig (*Surg., Gynec. and Obst.*, July 1932, 55, 35–44) shows the "cushion-like proliferation of the acinal wall" which corresponds to the picture I have set forth. Hellwig also (Endokrinologie, 1933, 12, 323–336) has discussed the differences between goiters in this country and abroad. Obviously the goiters in Germany differ from those in this country.

CHAPTER VI

Toxic Nodular Goiter

IN THE preceding chapter I tried to point out that even in the so-called nodular nontoxic stage there are elements already at work preparatory to the impending nodular toxic stage. Toxic, not because it is nodular, but in consequence of changes incident to the duration of the disease. In other words, the toxic nodular goiter is one that has reached a degree of toxicity which leaves no doubt about the advent of a state that is damaging the patient. It is a toxicity of degeneration and not of hyperplasia.

On the other hand, toxicity developing in a nodular nontoxic goiter may be associated with epithelial hyperplasia. These are the so-called Basedowified goiters of Kocher. In many cases both processes, toxicity of degeneration and thyrotoxicosis due to hyperplasia, co-exist. Toxicity due to degeneration usually may exist for a number of years until without known cause, the toxicity of hyperplasia, a true hypersecretion, is superimposed. In rare cases even a frank exophthalmic goiter is implanted on a nodular toxic goiter, just as it may be implanted on a diffuse or nontoxic goiter.

The toxic nodular is the most common goiter in the clinic. It bridges that indefinite gap between the diffuse nontoxic, or the nodular nontoxic goiter, and the degenerative goiter associated with goiter heart. In this sense it is an intermediate step to a more serious state. The importance of recognizing this lies in the fact that the surgeon is dealing with a condition which tends to become more serious than the one existing at the time of operation. It is not so much what it is as what it inevitably will become.

In the past a toxic goiter was viewed merely as one in which there was an excess of secretion, an over-functioning of the acinal epithelium. Since we appreciate more fully the relation of old goiters to heart disturbances it is necessary to recognize the toxicity of degeneration. When toxicity due to degeneration prevails, the cardiac disturbances dominate, whereas in cases where cellular hyperplasia is the chief factor, the signs of thyrotoxicosis are in evidence and reach a transcendent degree in exophthalmic goiter.

By keeping these two phases in mind, even though both are present, as is often the case, one can in the clinic predict the anatomic findings.

Conversely, the anatomic findings may aid in the interpretation of clinical signs which previously have not been clear.

From the foregoing it is obvious why it is most difficult to harmonize the laboratory findings in this group with the clinical diagnosis. The goiter influences which are tending toward the goiter heart are not expressed in terms of epithelial proliferation but in terms of degeneration. The most obvious structural changes are found in the study of the colloid unassociated with evidence of cellular activity. In contrast with this are the thyrotoxic signs which are evidence of an overzealous thyroid and find expression in terms of cellular hyperplasia that results in newly developed acini and columnar epithelium.

Therefore, before we can hope for harmony between the clinical and the laboratory findings, both groups of evidence need to be considered conjointly with full realization that evidence from both sources is necessary to a full understanding of the concrete case. Signs due to degeneration and those due to cellular hyperplasia must be accurately distinguished. This is usually possible in the clinic but histologic study must write the final conclusion. Even when given the most careful thought the problem is so complicated that there will be cases in which a difference of opinion must continue to exist. Pathologists have been prone, when the surgeon reported as toxic cases in which evidence of cell hyperplasia was lacking, to abandon attempts to harmonize the clinical and the pathologic. This confusion is clarified if degenerative changes are sought for, but there cannot be complete understanding if only a part of the evidence is considered.

Recognition of the advent of toxicity of either type, it was noted, depends largely on the experience and viewpoint of the observer. The need obviously is not only to recognize the toxicity in its earlier stages but also to ascertain which type of toxicity is responsible for the symptoms. It is clinically necessary to push the recognition of the beginning of the toxic state back to an earlier date and to determine whether it is expressive of degeneration or hyperplasia.

The necessity for earlier recognition has been emphasized since the need was admitted of removing colloid goiters, even in the supposedly nontoxic stage, because of the certain future development of a cardiotoxic state. This view has been forced on us because it is an every day experience to have patients vociferously proclaim how much better they feel since a goiter was removed, in cases of dubious toxicity. The obvious conclusion is that since the goiter must be operated on when it becomes toxic, it is wise to anticipate the more advanced stage and remove the lesion before more serious complications develop. It is the surgeon's business to relieve the patient of an incipient toxicity just as much as it is to relieve him of an incipient malignant tumor. Though often slow in its development, goiter in the end is a deadly disease.

In years gone one surgeon hesitated to operate on goiters which were only slightly toxic because when operated on at this period, patients returned years later with a new, generally more toxic, goiter. Now that we know that we can and must remove these early toxic goiters so completely that there will be no return, there no longer is hesitancy in operating in the early toxic stage.

The final tandem end of the nontoxic and the toxic goiter, uniform or nodular, is the goiter heart, that state in which the toxicity of the goiter is overshadowed by disturbance of the heart described in the next chapter. Here, likewise, it is difficult to determine when the terminal heart condition begins. Starting with the slight cardiac acceleration of the nontoxic goiters through the obviously toxic state and terminating in death from cardiac failure—that is the life history. With the first increase in the heart rate, in the so-called nontoxic nodular, the heart has sampled the first exhilarating cocktail which ultimately ends in delirium tremens expressed in arrhythmia and broken compensation.

In a careful clinical study of these cases one can very frequently follow the sequence of the symptoms. The patient may experience repeated crises to be followed by remissions. These may be endured until the cardiac complications become great enough to disable the patient. For this reason the basal rate can never have much, even theoretical, value in determining the mischief this type of goiter produces.

As a matter of fact most patients with toxic nodular goiter come, not because of the toxic symptoms, but because of an indefinite heart disturbance, which in its next stage will be a goiter heart. Too often, as noted above, we assume the patient's apprehension is due to a thyrotoxic state. Even now such patients, lacking an increased basal metabolic rate, are improperly diagnosed and operation is deferred in just those cases which require it most.

Formerly most goiter patients came because of a failing heart. The patient likely had been told years before that she had a goiter which was wholly innocent. The majority of goiter patients I saw thirty and more years ago were so interpreted; the thyroid had nothing to do with the complaints so far as either the patient or her doctor knew. Of the relation of this sign to the goiter she was no more ignorant than I; we both drank out of the same trough of prevailing medical opinion.

On the other hand, nowadays a patient is apt to be thyrotoxic-conscious and if anything goes wrong the goiter is blamed and her doctor is too prone to fall in with the suggestion. Removal of a goiter for nervous states wholly unrelated to toxic goiter must fail to produce the anticipated relief. Operation will relieve only such symptoms as are caused by the goiter.

The cases which are now most common in the clinic, however, are aware of an increased nervousness, loss of weight and usually increased weakness. These prodromal symptoms may continue for a considerable number of years before the patient is incapacitated or even seriously sick. So true is this that the secondary toxic adenomas, now the nodular toxic goiters, formerly said to begin most commonly at 15 to 20 years after the first discovery of the goiter, are now recognized at a much earlier period. This calendar calculation was a useful guide in years past but it holds no longer.

Many show symptoms of epithelial hyperplasia, besides nervousness, marked loss of weight and tremor. These signs may regress only to experience renewed exacerbations months or years later. Cases which improve and relapse, one may be sure, are associated with hyperplasia. Toxicity of degeneration, on the other hand, progresses uniformly. The history of the case therefore may aid much in predicting the anatomic findings.

Not all cases progress so leisurely. In the more severe cases the onset of toxicity may be so abrupt that within weeks or months a state is reached which renders operation hazardous. Even worse, the symptoms may be so stormy that the nature of the disease is not recognized and death ensues within a few weeks; or the goiter may be evident but the intensity of the symptoms render an operation impossible, or at least lead us to think so.

These stormy exacerbations may, as noted in the preceding chapter, be implanted on a goiter of minimal toxicity, or happen in cases in which the previous existence of a goiter is not recognized. Such cases commonly present cellular hyperplasia added to a pre-existing degenerating goiter. In the hyperacute it is common to find hyperplasia, the cells of which have degenerated even to the degree of exfoliation. These cases are not common but they are so frequent that the mortality from them is greater than that from operation in all other cases.

To summarize: in secondary toxic goiters degeneration or hyperplasia may be present and in many cases they are associated. Whichever is present the final stage is a degenerated goiter which results in goiter heart.

Pathogenesis. A renewed confession of ignorance regarding the cause of goiter does not belong here. That belongs to its incestive periods. This chapter has to do with something already on the way. The duty here is to conduct it through this division, as the railroad men say.

As has been previously stated, what we mean by a toxic nodular goiter is merely one in which the degree of disturbance has reached a point where the removal of the disease is demanded. We do not mean that the

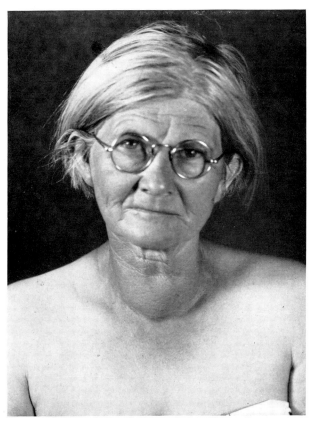

FIG. 90. Toxic colloid goiter. Age 54. Goiter since childhood. Nervous, short of breath, pulse 120. Thyroid uniformly enlarged, hard. The thyroid caused a uniform moderate protrusion.

goiter previously was not at all toxic, only that the damage it did was tolerable. In other words, whatever boosted the adolescent goiter into a nontoxic nodular pushed it another stage ahead into a toxic nodular. Nothing new has come into the picture, except a flag station for the through train to whistle at, not for.

If the goiter was known to exist before the onset of the toxic symptoms one may say without equivocation that it is a secondary toxic one.

If the enlargement of the thyroid gland was nodulated or of markedly unequal size on the two sides, particularly if the patient is in midlife, we can safely say that it is a toxic nodular goiter whether it is obviously nodular or not. This is important to note because the toxic diffuse, of the accepted nomenclature, differs usually in the rapidity of its onset, its more common occurrence in earlier years and the lesser cardiac compli-

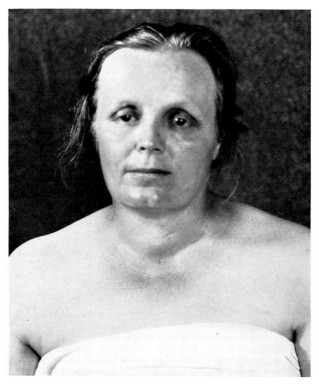

FIG. 91. Toxic colloid goiter. Age 45. Goiter 15 years. Nervous the past five years. Some loss of weight the last few weeks. Pulse 136. Definitely nodular goiter.

cations. However, this state may be engrafted on either the nontoxic or the toxic nodular.

From the foregoing it is plain that the advent of the toxic stage, following the nontoxic, may present a varying picture, depending much on the rapidity of onset and the degree attained. In all cases the patient is sick of her goiter as well as sick from it. Because of the varying picture these goiters present it is impossible to discuss them satisfactorily in an abstract way. Each runs a different course, and to appreciate the various factors one must study the patient, as well as the slide, both before and after the operation. Much that one finds has its analogy in the nontoxic stage because it is a matter of a quantitative not a qualitative change. Since different persons react differently to the same stimuli, the reaction of different patients will differ in correspondence to degrees of structural variation. Goiters vary in histology in the divers parts, hence a

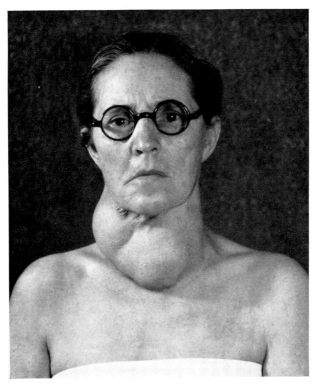

Fig. 92. Nodular toxic goiter, patient aged 60. Duration of goiter 30 years. Weight loss 40 pounds, pulse 125, heart fast for 5 years. Goiter freely movable.

repeated study of the specimen may be required in order to find what is dominant.

Just how the toxic stage of the nodular goiter is reached is a complicated question. Before the generally recognized stage of toxicity is reached there often is periodic appearance of evidences of toxicity, followed by periods when this sign is in abeyance or absent. As previously noted, it is unlikely any two observers would be in entire agreement as to when the toxic stage has been reached.

Naturally, pathologists scoff at the idea of determining the nature of the pathologic lesion by inspecting the patient. Nevertheless, one may gain very valuable information just by looking at the patient. Of course, information gained by inspection is only suggestive, but it sometimes serves as a criterion for checking other evidence. This is particularly useful if we have observed the patient from time to time over a period of years as it makes a comparison with previous states possible.

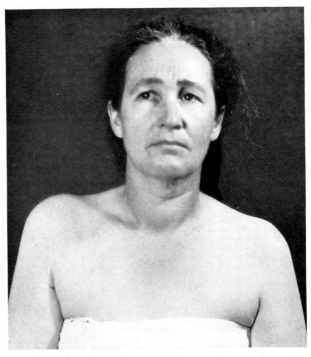

FIG. 93. Nodular toxic goiter. Age 44. The tense features bespeak a suppressed nervousness. Pulse 110, loss of 25 pounds in 8 months.

We may begin by discussing a small goiter, apparently uniform on inspection (Fig. 90). The face of the patient is wrinkled and prematurely aged. Though the goiter is of some years' duration the nodulations may be apparent, but its long duration allows us to judge that it belongs to this group and that it is really a nodular toxic in all clinical essentials; a cross-section will show it to be such anatomically. The toxicity is not apparent; there is no evident nervousness; loss of weight and a rapid heart are all the clinic has to show. Yet it would be a gross error to regard these as belonging to an earlier and a simpler stage.

In other cases the irregularity of the gland is not apparent on inspection but is definitely proved by palpation. Naturally the nodulations are less easily discerned, due to increase of adipose tissue in the neck. This is particularly true in the submyxedemic (Fig. 91). Complaisance rather than tension characterizes the facial expression of this type.

Those in whom the progress to toxicity is slow, particularly those in whom the nodulations are so large that they are pendulous, may show

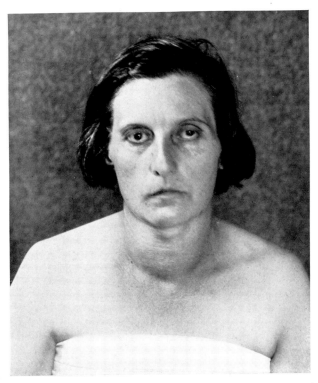

FIG. 94. Toxic nodular goiter. Age 35. Goiter four years. Lost 30 pounds in weight, pulse 130. Goiter slightly nodulated and hard.

very little evidence of toxicity. The loss of weight is likely to be considerable, but being spread over a number of years the patient is not greatly incapacitated nor concerned thereby (Fig. 92).

Some of these patients have a fixed gaze, sometimes a widened palpebral fissure, and the intern is liable to register positive eye signs. These are typical of a numerous group who complain of minor nervousness. There may be neither loss of weight, nor notable cardiac disturbance

(Fig. 93). These patients are prone to complain little but their families are likely to sense a tense state.

Those most frequently overlooked are the depressed type (Fig. 94). They complain of nothing in particular, but the facial expression reflects

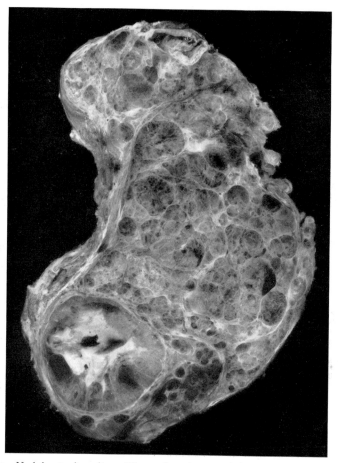

FIG. 95. Nodular toxic goiter. The surface is smooth but the cross-section shows many small nodules well encapsulated. Below a degenerating fetal adenoma. Age 62. Goiter 30 years. Pulse 140.

the mental state. The loss of weight and the rapid heart are apt to be regarded as secondary. Frequently even the presence of goiter is overlooked—or ignored if it is discovered.

In contrast with the above are the more acute toxic states engrafted on nodular toxic goiter. The milder cases show the somewhat apprehen-

sive look of the more acutely toxic. More pronounced cases may display
all the manifestations of the primary acute toxic goiter that will be described in the chapter on Graves' disease. This type is more frequently
engrafted on the earlier adolescent or nontoxic cases than on the toxic.
These are the Basedowified goiters of Kocher. They present the manifestations of the more acute primary disease: the agitated appearance,
the obvious nervousness, the hyperemia, and in extreme cases even an

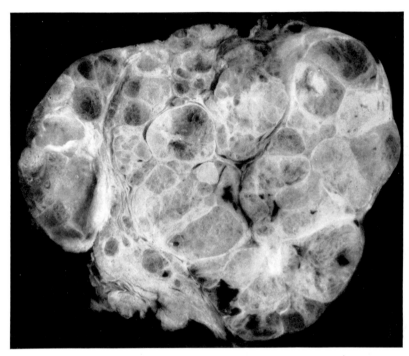

Fɪɢ. 96. Toxic adenoma. The lobulations show dark areas with lighter centers with
some small cysts.

exophthalmos. There is this difference between them and the primarily
acutely toxic: heart manifestations of a serious nature are more apt to
appear, particularly in the early days following operation. The long
existing old colloid goiter has, in the intervening years, done something
to the heart which may not be apparent until after the operation. These
represent cases in the stage preceding definite signs of thyrotoxic heart.
These cases are much less likely than the primary toxic type to lessen
their degree of toxicity and enter a more quiescent state. The secondary
Basedow's usually continue in a severely toxic state indefinitely, and

when engrafted on a case in which the heart is notably affected spontaneous death is the probable outcome.

Because of the long duration of many of these goiters one may find the most weird combinations of symptoms. One wonders what the goiter is trying to do. Symptoms of degenerated toxic, some of hyperplastic toxic are each trying to find clinical expression. This is particularly impressive when associated with thyrotoxicosis and myxedema presenting symptoms more or less significant of each. Naturally such cases present complicated pictures in the laboratory and cannot be classified in any

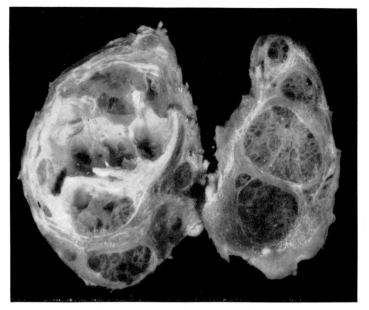

FIG. 97. Toxic nodular goiter. Age 24. Goiter 6 years. Lost 30 pounds. Right lobe largely cystic, the left contains many large cystic acini.

one group for the simple reason that the several areas represent several groups anatomically as well as clinically.

Pathology. The external form of these goiters obviously does not differ essentially from the nontoxic because they are such with something added.

The pathological study of these goiters must begin in the clinic. The glands are firmer to palpation than the nontoxic goiters. When only slightly toxic they are freely movable on the surrounding tissues, but the more acutely toxic may be more or less firmly fixed. This fixity and sensitiveness to pressure are usually accurate measures of toxicity.

At the operating table the capsule is found to be adherent to the covering structures; the veins are larger, the whole gland redder in color and on the whole firmer. If the capsule of the nodules is ruptured the contents pour forth as a granular mass.

Like the nontoxic, these goiters may be uniform in superficial outline (Fig. 95) and yet have all the clinical and anatomic characteristics of the nodulated. Even large nodulations on section may present a uniform superficial outline.

The typically nodular toxic goiter is made up of sizable nodules en-

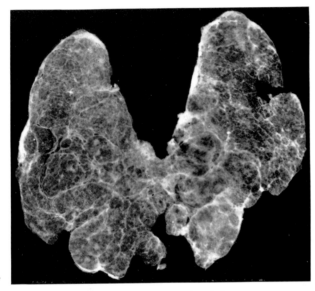

FIG. 98. Toxic colloid goiter. Age 24. Nervous breakdown two years ago. On admission pulse was 85. The gland was hard and at operation friable and very adherent.

closed in definite capsule-like structures. The less toxic have a whitish almost translucent color indistinguishable grossly from the nontoxic, but as the condition advances hemorrhagic areas appear (Fig. 96). Cyst-like areas are not uncommon, particularly in those of long duration (Fig. 97), which are prone to protrude even to the extent of becoming pendent. In these cases, even after operation and laboratory examinations, one awaits the after-course in order to determine just how much the goiter really disturbed the patient.

In those cases in which the advent of toxicity is more abrupt, usually in younger patients presenting moderate nodulosity, the cut surface is mottled grayish red (Fig. 98). The grayish areas represent areas of maximum hyperplasia. Generally the more aggravated the toxicity, the more these resemble the diffuse toxic goiters, true Graves' disease.

Varying degrees and types of degeneration may be observed. Calcareous degeneration is not uncommon in the aged but represents a terminal state. Cystic areas may occupy a considerable part of the gland. The more cystic, the less toxic as a rule. These degenerations are not a part of the toxic gland. Sometimes the cysts have papillary projections into their lumina which are occasionally mistaken for the papillations of Graves' disease (Fig. 99).

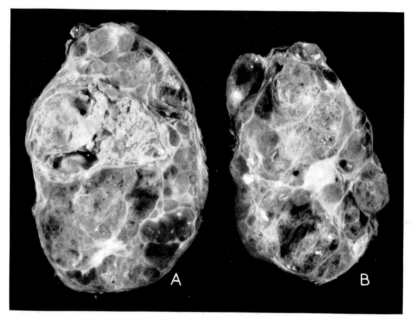

FIG. 99. Toxic nodular goiter. Age 53. *A*, irregular calcareous area in the center. *B*, Area of fibrosis in the center.

Histology. In order to harmonize the microscopic findings with the clinical signs one must distinguish between two classes of changes, the degenerative and the hyperplastic.

The slowly developing toxicity on the nontoxic nodular goiter is naturally one of degree. In the early cases the acinal hyperplasia of the toxic is not impressive (*A*, Fig. 100), being the same as the nontoxic save that there is more acinal proliferation. The average size of the acinal cells with more deeply staining nuclei (*B*, Fig. 100) is all that is apparent. Sometimes there is little to account for the increased nervousness ob-

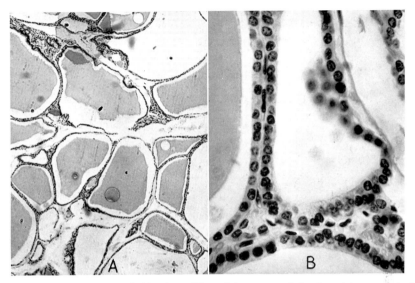

FIG. 100. Early toxic colloid goiter. The acini vary much in size with many small ones between the larger ones. *A,* Low power showing the proportionate number of the small acini. *B,* The epithelium is cuboid in some of the smaller acini and more deeply staining. The colloid is variously dense.

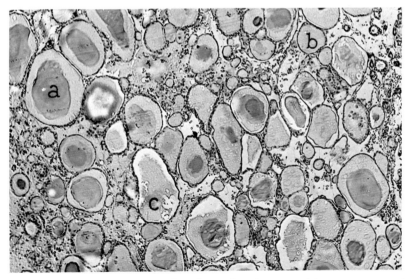

FIG. 101. Nodular toxic goiter. The cells are flat, degenerated in some areas; *a,* the colloid is basophilic in the center with a rim of acidophilic about the border; *b,* a few are acidophilic; *c,* in some areas the colloid is degenerated.

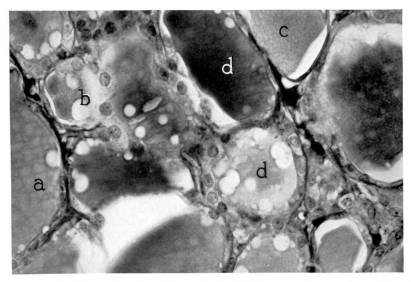

Fig. 102. Nodular toxic goiter with marked colloid degeneration: *a*, acinus with cellular atrophy; *b*, large cells in a state of degeneration; *c*, granular colloid; *d,d*, variously staining colloid. The colloid in most acini shows retraction and other evidence of degeneration.

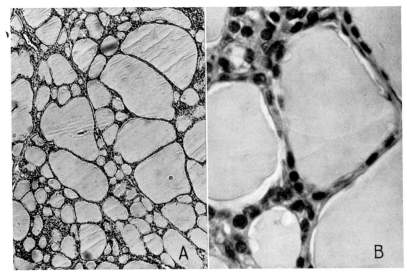

Fig. 103. Nodular toxic goiter: *A*, low power showing little change in epithelium or colloid. *B*, Same, high power, in which some acini show cell atrophy, even to disappearance. The colloid stains irregularly and shows degeneration. There are masses of cells between the acini in both pictures.

served in the clinic. In such cases two possibilities must be considered: the patient may have overestimated the disturbance, or the trouble may lie elsewhere. However, in these cases evidence of degeneration must be sought for. The first changes are to be found in the colloid. Instead of staining with eosin it stains with hematoxylin; that is to say, the colloid has become basophilic (Fig. 101). In some cases the change may not be apparent when stained with eosin (*A*, Fig. 101) but is revealed when stained with methylene blue (*B*, Fig. 101). What these changes mean in terms of chemistry is not known. The early changes do not respond to

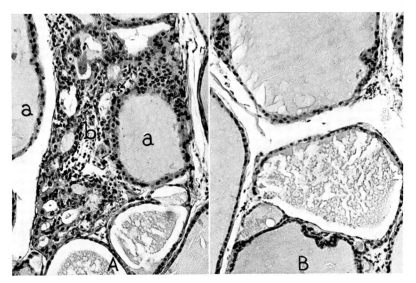

Fig. 104. Newly formed acini in an old colloid goiter: *A,a,a,* old acini with flat epithelium and markedly degenerated colloid; *b,* newly formed acini with cuboidal well staining epithelium; *B,* old acini lined with flat and degenerated cells. The colloid is faintly staining and granular.

hematoxylin but do to more delicate tests, notably Mallory's aniline blue. When more pronounced the eosin stains with hematoxylin. This relationship becomes obvious only when both stains are used on the same tissue. It should be noted also that different areas of a goiter may show great variations, whereupon more than one block of tissue should be examined. The presence of these changes accounts for notable degrees of toxicity in the absence of cell proliferation. It is the toxicity of early degeneration, not that of hyperplasia.

In more pronounced toxic cases the colloid changes are more obvious. The tinctorial changes progress to the stage of degeneration (Fig. 102). The colloid stains irregularly, some palely, some not at all, with an admixture of these and densely staining areas all in the same acinus. Associated with these is cell atrophy and degeneration. What is of greater interest is the presence of large cells with palely staining or degenerated protoplasm. They resemble the cell changes in Hashimoto's struma and are prone to be followed by postoperative myxedema.

Areas showing the above changes may form only a part of the goiter while the greater area shows a more simple structure which in low power may be quite unimpressive (*A*, Fig. 103). Closer examination shows cell

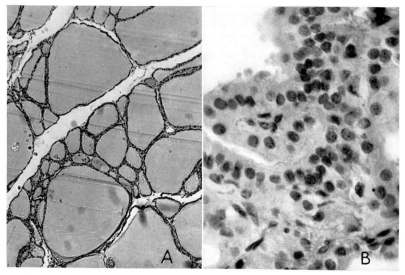

Fig. 105. Nodular toxic goiter with beginning acinal hyperplasia. *A*, Nontoxic area showing small and large acini. *B*, Toxic area. The cells are columnar, the nuclei large and well staining. In some areas the cells are disarranged. The colloid is sharply defined.

atrophy and degeneration and colloid which stains irregularly (*B*, Fig. 103).

In some cases, in addition to the tinctorial change in the colloid, there are newly formed acini, either within the interspaces or within the walls of the old acini showing a taller and an obviously more active epithelium (Fig. 104). Some small areas show a greater activity (Fig. 105). Even though the greater part of the gland exhibits a state parallel with the nontoxic, these small areas of hyperplasia represent mild clinical evidence of hyperplastic toxicity. In such cases the acini in the interacinal spaces only show an increased activity while the epithelium lining the old acini remains flat as above noted (Fig. 106). In others all the acini partake in hypertrophy, still other areas in hyperplasia (Fig. 107). These are usually

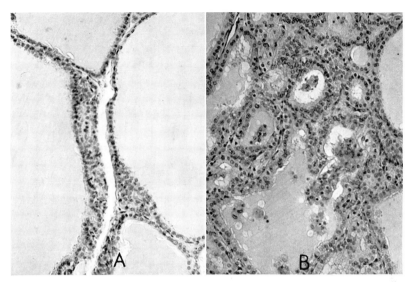

Fig. 106. Secondary Graves' disease implanted on a nodular toxic goiter: *A*, area showing but slight hyperplasia; *B*, typical papillations of exophthalmic goiter extending into the lumina of the acini. The colloid is in the main well staining. There is some cell exfoliation.

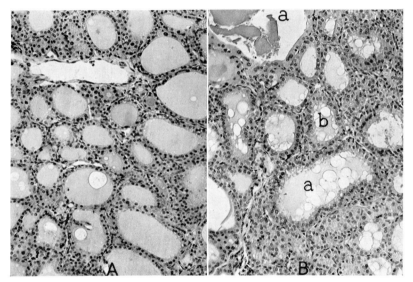

Fig. 107. Toxic nodular goiter of the acute type: *A*, hypertrophy of the acinal epithelium in the nontoxic area; *B*, besides the hypertrophy of the old acini, *a,a*, there is a definite hyperplasia at *b*. Many newly formed acini contain no colloid being represented only by cell masses.

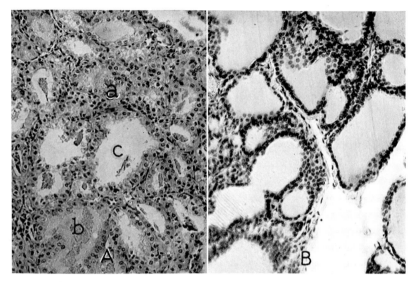

FIG. 108. Very toxic nodular goiter showing cell degeneration: *A*,*a*, acini showing cell degeneration; *b*, granular colloid; *c*, acini with stainless colloid; *B*, area of the goiter not notably affected in the acute hyperplasia, but the colloid is faintly staining.

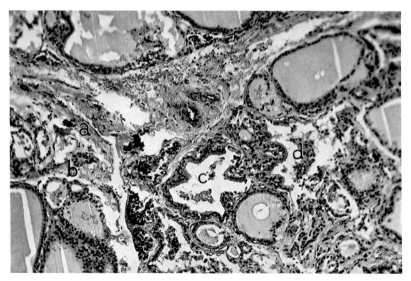

FIG. 109. Nodular toxic goiter with degeneration: *a*, area of degenerated fibrosis; *b*, degeneration of cells in areas not involved in hyperplasia; *c*, well preserved hyperplastic cells; *d*, the same in a state of degeneration. The colloid represents many states of stainability.

found in younger patients and present a step toward true Graves' disease. Those on which a Basedow have become implanted of course show the characteristic papillations.

In very toxic states there may be evidence of degeneration characterized by pronounced colloid changes (*A*, Fig. 108), even to the degeneration of the acinal cells. Other areas present simple cell hyperplasia with colloid changes (*B*, Fig. 108). Usually the simpler changes make up the bulk of the goiter and careless examination may miss the more important changes entirely.

In the hypertoxic, which occur most commonly in long existing goiters, toxic or not, seen most commonly in women beyond the menopause, the changes are more pronounced. In addition to the signs of degeneration incident to age of both goiter and patient there is evidence of further changes. There may be evidence of epithelial proliferation which in turn has degenerated. The toxicity of the newly formed cells seem to have resulted in their own degeneration (Fig. 109). This sort of change is most commonly observed in those who die after a short stormy period of hyperpyrexia and delirium.

Literature

Secondary Toxic Goiter. There is no literature which attempts to explain how the allegedly nontoxic goiter becomes toxic except those in which a secondary Graves' disease is implanted on a previous colloid. How or why this happens literature is as silent as the slide. The slide holds some promise of explanation, the literature nothing. That there is a progressive change from the simple to the toxic colloid is generally recognized as noted by Hinton (*Ann. Surg.*, April 1932, 95, 499–502) and Hertzler (*Arch. Surg.*, 1928, 16, 61). Enzer (*Ann. Int. Med.*, June 1930, 3, 1241–1251) makes a noteworthy attempt to bring some order out of chaos but the presentation is a bit deep for a surgeon.

CHAPTER VII

The Cardiotoxic Goiter

BY A cardiotoxic goiter is meant one that causes a disturbance of the heart due to a toxic substance released by degenerative changes in the goiter. It is always associated with some changes in the colloid the nature of which is not known. Not knowing what it is we must confine our attention to what it does. That the substance released by the degeneration acts on the heart in the beginning as only an irritant is evidenced by the fact that if the source of the poison is removed by thyroidectomy the heart quickly returns to normal and remains so. But a time comes when this salutory return to normal does not follow removal of the goiter, and we may then conclude that there are associated degenerative changes in the heart muscle itself though the anatomic evidence is not convincing.

In preceding chapters it was stressed that it is necessary in toxic goiters to distinguish between the toxicity of hyperplasia and that of degeneration. The cardiotoxic goiter is associated with only the degenerated, never with the hyperplastic goiter. True a typical hyperplastic goiter, as exemplified by Graves' disease, ultimately dies a cardiotoxic death, but only after hyperplasia gives way to degeneration.

There is no definite cellular pathology in the cardiotoxic goiter nor are there definite changes on the part of the heart. In the study of the disease we can determine a definite disturbance of the heart only in the clinic, and by its sequellae. We can view the goiter after thyroidectomy and see what it looks like. In the same ultimate heart failure we can subject the heart muscle to a similar scrutiny. Fortunately it is now possible to study the effect of the goiter on the heart by a total thyroidectomy in all stages of the disease, thus at once determining the effect it has had on the heart and at the same time securing material for histologic study. The obvious conclusion is that the goiter was responsible for the cardiac condition. By the laboratory study of the tissue thus removed and by finding a constant change the demands of scientific investigations are fulfilled, at least for clinical purposes.

It cannot be too often repeated that all goiters beyond early adult life are cardiotoxic to a greater or lesser degree. Everything imports that when once hyperplasia of the thyroid epithelium has begun, the road has been opened to a cardiotoxic end, however long it may be before

130

the heart symptoms dominate the right of way. This is indicated by the increase in pulse rate, an inevitable concomitant of even the nontoxic stage. We have to deal in this chapter with that stage of the thyroid disease in which the cardiac symptoms become prominent. At this stage the goiter, whether toxic or not, assumes a secondary rôle as far as the clinician is concerned.

The study of the pathology therefore has a definite purpose: namely, to determine the relation of the pathologic changes in the thyroid gland to certain heart symptoms. Such a study brings a full appreciation that although goiters are not thyrotoxic yet they are not "innocent." Furthermore, the relation of the thyroid gland, independent of goitrous enlargement, to the cardiac state is just beginning to excite interest. It is possible that the cardiac effect is produced, not because the goiter is degenerating, but because the thyroid gland is degenerating, as the result of involutional changes.

Naturally the cases in which the heart is a dominating factor have various degrees of severity: early, well advanced, terminal. In the early cases there usually is more or less toxic goiter, degenerative or hyperplastic; the heart condition is but incidental, since the removal of the goiter, by eliminating the heart irritant produced by the goiter, relieves the heart permanently. This is the most striking result the surgeon can achieve. In the more advanced cases the heart lesion is a real factor and demands removal of the goiter regardless of whether it is toxic in its own right or not. The goiter—it may or may not be or have been toxic—as such is of purely secondary concern. It is the heart disturbance that demands relief. In the terminal stage, as the term indicates, the disease has advanced until the removal of a goiter is either impossible or of no avail.

In studying the structure of the goiters associated with cardiac disturbances we may divide them into the following groups: those in which the cardiac signs disappear after removal of the goiter; those in which a cardiac death follows operation; and those in which a cardiac death is not preceded by operation.

In days gone by unless a goiter produced toxicity, supposedly a hyperfunction, it was called nontoxic, which was equivalent to exonerating it of all blame. The result of this viewpoint was that surgeons confined their efforts to the removal of a sufficient amount of the goiter to relieve what was thought to be the thyrotoxic symptoms. This done the ideal end of surgery was believed to have been attained. That the residuum might become cardiotoxic was not considered. Our surgical philosophy, like our theology, is made to meet the demands of the state of our knowledge. The fetish "cachexia thyreopriva" of Kocher has for more than fifty years frightened operators into leaving an arbitrary portion of the gland at the operation. It now transpires that in our fear of removing too much we left enough to degenerate and produce in the course of years a goiter heart.

Only after it was discovered that the dire results foretold by Kocher did not follow total removal of the gland in adults was it possible to relieve the heart by a very radical thyroidectomy. As so often happens in surgery when it is discovered that something can be done, abundant reasons are at hand for doing it; so having discovered that even complete removal of the thyroid gland could be done, very radical operations or even complete 'ectomies were at once in order. Fortunately this revelation was vouchsafed at a time when goiter's baneful effect on the heart was coming to be recognized. Nothing is more pleasing to the surgical fraternity than to discover simultaneously the technical possibility of an operation and an indication calling for it. Nowhere in surgery is there to be found a happier example of such a coincidence.

Following the practice of other writers of serial stories it seems advisable to present here a brief synopsis of the events recounted in the preceding chapters: In early life the thyroid gland attempts to adjust itself to function harmoniously with the other endocrine glands; or, partaking too much or too little of something, it becomes the colloid goiter of adolescence. There being no anatomic change, spontaneous recovery is possible. If the enlargement does not regress with the passage of time the goiter changes its shape, developing nontoxic bosselations. During this period neither patient nor doctor can quite decide whether the goiter is toxic or not, and in their combined optimism they regard it as nontoxic. Then follows the chapter when everybody learns that the goiter is toxic— nodular toxic—and there is a scurrying to do something about it.

It is obvious that we must go back much farther than has been our wont in studying the effect of goiter on the heart. Old bosselated goiters, supposedly innocent throughout life, are actually constantly at work. The so-called nontoxic nodular goiters frequently pass directly to a cardiotoxic state without there having been compelling evidence of thyroid toxicity, in the ordinary sense, at any period of the disease. Let it be repeated that absence of thyrotoxic manifestations does not attest that the heart is not being injured by the goiter. A slight increase in pulse rate and some nervousness now and then are unlikely to cause great concern in the minds of either patient or doctor until a failing heart compels recognition of the baneful effect of the goiter.

True, the majority of cases give indubitable evidence of thyrotoxicosis, nodular toxic or uniform, as the case may be, at some period during their course. Yet a considerable proportion of patients who come to the clinic because of impaired health are unaware of the presence of thyroid disease. Because the goiter is small and the general symptoms of nervousness are indefinite (perhaps some loss of weight), the cardiac disturbance is not ascribed to the goiter even though an enlargement is discovered. These cases are purely degenerative; neither hyperplasia nor thyrotoxic is considered, in the sense of hyperthyroidism, as having ever played a part.

Even the more acute diffuse goiter characterized by epithelial hyperplasia, with or without eye signs, loses its toxicity after a time, but slumbers on and sooner or later develops degeneration, identical with that of degenerative toxic glands. And the heart suffers, not because of the hyperplasia, but because of the degeneration which accompanies or follows it. Thus the finale of a Graves' disease, just as certainly as that of colloid goiter, is a cardiac death. I have observed a number of such cases in which the goiter "burned out" and the cardiac death was delayed more than 30 years. I have under observation now a patient who nearly 40 years ago had an acute exophthalmic goiter of such a severe character that delirium and high fever attended it. Complete regression of all symptoms save the exophthalmos followed, but in recent years cardiac symptoms have become manifest—and of the ultimate end I have not the slightest doubt.

More treacherous still are those thyroid processes which, never reaching the clinical dignity of goiter, undergo changes that attract the attention of neither patient nor doctor until cardiopathies start both in search of the cause. The clinical history is easy enough to trace when a palpable goiter is in evidence; but when a goiter has not been discovered or as much as suspected, even after the cardiac symptoms have become evident, the case is disconcerting. Sometimes it is necessary to diagnose a goiter heart from the nature of the general symptoms, coupled with the character of the cardiac disturbances, and then proceed to operation even though the thyroid is not palpable. These cases are the surgeon's delight.

Caution needs to be exercised lest we regard such thyroids as normal and the associated lesion of the heart as primary or idiopathic. The fact that there is no epithelial hyperplasia cannot be construed as evidence that the thyroid is normal. It is imperative in such cases that one study the histochemistry of the colloid. That arteriosclerotic cardiac diseases are influenced by the total ablation of the thyroid gland may be admitted, but that this is due to the removal of a normal gland has not been proved.

The goiter having gone through the many stages above noted ere reaching the cardiotoxic stage, the question arises, what record have these left on the structure of the thyroid gland? Although each stage may leave its trace, it is impossible for the pathologist to write a story accurately describing the clinical course of all cases because no two of them run parallel in rate, time or degree. It requires the combined knowledge of the clinic, the operating room and the laboratory, and even the life history of the patient after operation for even an approximately complete depictment. To add to the labor and exasperation of the pathologist some of the hieroglyphics of the disease are written in one part of the gland, some in another, consequently an extended laboratory study may be necessary to bring some semblance of order out of chaos. The study of a single block of tissue may be misleading, and dependence on a simple routine stain even more so. Certain it is that one must study each case as an entity, comparing the various anatomic changes with the clinical signs.

In our present state of knowledge, or ignorance, it seems impossible to formulate a working hypothesis. The only consistent change is in the histochemistry of the colloid. This being the constant factor it is reasonable to assume that degeneration of the colloid is responsible.

The less impressive cases in which cardiac irregularities and general evidence of decompensation develop during a period of months or years even without toxic symptoms likewise indicate that degeneration and not the hyperplasia is the essential factor. These cases, which run a leisurely course with little sign of cardiac disturbance, suddenly manifest hyperplastic toxicity, even to the degree of true Basedow's disease, and as the slide shows hyperplasia, one may be misled into believing that this is the essential feature. Yet the colloid changes are present and the evidence is that they have been present for a long time.

These cases suggest that the heart is being constantly overdosed with a substance which does not cause anatomic changes in the heart muscle. This group, having gradually developed cardiac symptoms, suddenly shows acute exacerbation of the heart rate and irregularities as though poisoned by a drug. This is particularly notable in old Basedow patients who, having burned out and remained in fair health, even for decades, suddenly develop alarming cardiac symptoms. Epithelial hyperplasia is commonly found in such cases, which suggests that the hyperplasia whipped up a failing heart with fatal results.

Most of the operative deaths occur in patients who have an affected heart which is indicated by alterations in rate and rhythm. Chief importance attaches to the duration of the cardiac manifestations rather than to the degree of disturbance. The deaths are due to cardiac failure. There may be no unfavorable constitutional manifestations whatever. In most cases the heart seems to fag out; the rate increases, the force lessens. This end is most likely to follow in patients who have taken Lugol's solution for a long time. This drug apparently expedites colloidal changes which are regularly associated with goiter heart. The clinic attests the fact that these changes are permanent. Their postoperative course is unpredictable. No period of preoperative care has any subsequent influence in these Lugolized patients.

As noted above, changes in the colloid are the only constant feature in cardiotoxic goiters. One finds a play of colors in the colloid as various dyes are used and this is referred to in general terms as basophilic colloid. Lacking a chemical formula one can only speak in terms of tinctorial chemistry. It would seem there is a chemical change in the colloid which results in the formation of some cardiotoxic substance. In this respect the changes are the same as those discussed in connection with toxic nodular goiters. The final heart failure is but a summation of those processes.

Cases which present themselves in a final state which forbids operation or in which any procedure is hazardous form a separate group. In addition to the usual signs of secondary toxicity such as were described in the previous chapter, there are signs of heart failure indicated by dyspnea and dropsy.

The most extreme cases may present high fever and intense nervous reactions to the point of wild delirium. These have an added anatomic peculiarity in that the cells stain badly, or not at all, and areas show desquamation of epithelium. Whether these evidences represent an added pathologic process or if it is a terminal state is difficult to say.

By studying each case individually and by employing every means of both laboratory and clinic, we may hope to accumulate a set of figures which may eventually add up to something.

Pathogenesis. An attempt to study the genesis of the goiter heart in the clinic is beset with many difficulties due chiefly to the fact that we do not know what we are dealing with. We may assume that there are two processes at work. In one there is merely the stimulation by degenerative substances or by oversecretion which is seen in Graves' disease as noted in the previous chapter. The rapid rate can continue for many years without permanent damage. In the other process there is no notable disturbance of rate until the first symptoms are expressed in terms of disturbed rate and volume. We may assume this type to be due to some factor other than increased cell secretion.

As long as the heart remains regular in rate and volume there is no way of knowing whether it is suffering or not. The electrocardiograph has failed to give useful evidence. However, if the heart becomes intermittent in rate and volume, in the absence of evidence of organic heart disease, we must assume it is due to intoxication from the goiter. When evidences of decompensation develop we know for sure that the heart is failing; but, let it be noted, the presence of decompensation in the presence of a goiter does not make it a goiter heart. One must think of other possible causes of decompensation.

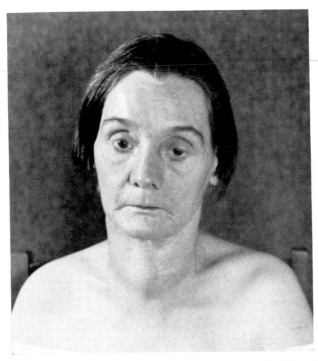

FIG. 110. Cardiotoxic goiter. Age 59. Dyspnea for 5 years of undetermined origin. Has known of goiter 22 years. Never was known to be toxic. Pulse 140, irregular in rate and volume.

Just how far back one needs to go to study the effect of the goiter on the heart it is difficult to say. One can learn much by observation of patients in the clinic. In the irritable heart sometimes associated with the simple goiter of adolescence their cheerful countenances dispose one to conclude that rapid hearts are of purely nervous origin. In the acutely toxic goiters allied with rapid heart the expression is apprehensive. Here also it may be that the heart is whipped up through the action of the controlling nerves. Sedatives and rest in bed may be followed by marked improvement in a very few days.

The cardiotoxic patient has a look of apprehension (Fig. 110). It differs from the expression of nervous excitation, just as the expression of a patient with cancer of the stomach differs from that of one who has a pylorospasm and fears he has a cancer. This is particularly true of patients who do not associate their trouble with a goiter, either because they

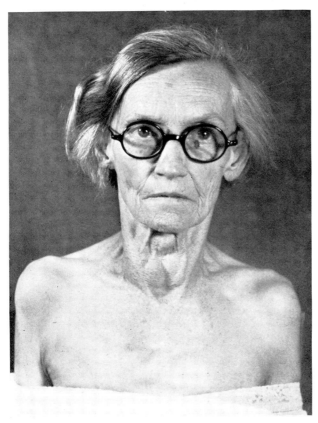

FIG. 111. Cardiotoxic goiter. Age 60. Had goiter 25 years. Gradually increasing cardiac irregularity, rate 150. Heart widely dilated.

regard the goiter as innocent or because they are unaware of the existence of any thyroid involvement. Those who have long had a toxic goiter with a rapid heart associate the two and accept the advancing heart trouble as a matter of course (Fig. 111). They are likely to have an associated loss of weight which is evident at a glance (Fig. 112). This loss of weight makes even the small goiter visible. All cases have in common an appearance of senility far beyond their years. The inelasticity of the skin emphasizes this fact. And, it may be added, that as surgical risks they rate their apparent age irrespective of their calendar age.

In the more advanced cases the increasing dyspnea may distort the facial expression by intensified distress and cyanosis.

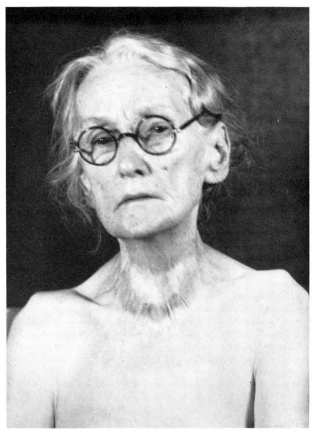

Fig. 112. Cardiotoxic goiter. Age 65. Goiter 37 years. Pulse 120, heart widely dilated and fibrillating.

That the heart disturbance in these cases is due to decompensation is attested by the fact that these patients, even when dropsical, may recuperate sufficiently by the use of sedatives and bed rest to make removal of the gland possible. That the condition is due, even in these stages of marked cardiac disturbance, to something the goiter continues to deliver to the patient is made evident by the fact that careful thyroidectomy allows the heart to return to an astonishing degree of efficiency.

Then follows the stage of complete decompensation with edema in the various tissues and cavities, but the face does not become edematous and this makes it possible to exclude other types of dropsy, notably that due to nephritis. These cases frequently become mentally confused due to disturbed circulation. There is lacking the violent delirium and hyperpyrexia of the terminal state. One curious feature of these cases is noteworthy: The violent terminal symptoms may be associated with a rapid reduction of the size of the goiter. This is apparently due to a rapid absorption of a destructive secretion.

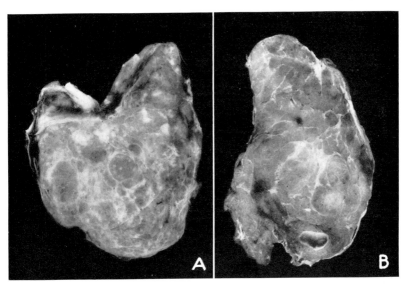

FIG. 113. Cardiotoxic thyroid. Patient died two days after operation: *A*, the right lobe was suffused, the outline of the various structures indistinct; *B*, the left lobe was that of an old chronic toxic goiter.

Pathology. The gross pathologic changes differ little from those of the two preceding stages, the nontoxic and the toxic nodular goiters. There is more evidence of fibrosis as one would expect because the patients generally are older. Since we have to do with a continuation of processes initiated in the preceding chapters it is self-evident that no striking innovations are to be expected here. We are concerned more with pathologic physiology than with pathologic anatomy.

The palpatory changes are dependent on the nature of the process. If there is recrudescence of the toxicity the gland is likely to be firm. If much fibrosed there likewise is increased density. The increased density is of prime importance in small goiters that are usually discovered during a search for a possible cause of cardiopathy; in fact it is distinctive. When a thyroid so small that it is barely palpable is dense to the touch we can identify it as the culprit we are seeking.

The first impressive pathologic change that confronts the surgeon is the friability of old colloid goiters when they are exposed at operation. The capsule tears easily and the parenchyma oozes out like brain tissue. It is usually reddish brown in color and the consistency of exuberant granulation tissue. This state of the fibrous tissue is usually due to degeneration, rarely to the acuteness of the glandular reaction. However,

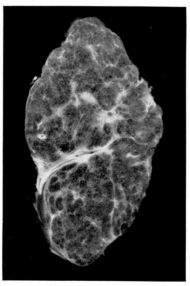

FIG. 114. Thyrotoxic goiter. Severe exophthalmic goiter 30 years before which burned out after a few years. Fair health 25 years, and died from cardiac failure.

these physical changes may be encountered in equal degree in toxic nodular goiters or even in the nontoxic, without notable cardiac change.

When the bosselated goiters become cardiotoxic the gross specimen does not differ from the simple toxic or even the nontoxic.

The small late-appearing goiters are different. The connective tissue is firm, the gland is inelastic and the vascularity is slight (Fig. 113). In burned-out Graves' disease when there is epithelial rejuvenation the surface may be brownish red (Fig. 114). Cases in which the existence of a goiter was not recognized until search was made for a possible explanation of a cardiac failure present a different picture. The thyroid is firm, sometimes so hard that cancer is simulated and may even be indistinguishable at the operating. These thyroids may be but little enlarged, and the term "cardiotoxic thyroid" is more exact anatomically than "cardiotoxic goiter."

Increasing study of this type of cardiotoxic cases with thyroids enlarged very little suggests the possibility that the thyroid gland may produce a cardiotoxic state without ever having become goitrous at all. There may be no notable physiologic disturbance, as in simple colloid goiter of adolescence; no notable epithelial proliferation, as in toxic goiter. The thymus starts our development, atrophies in a few years and

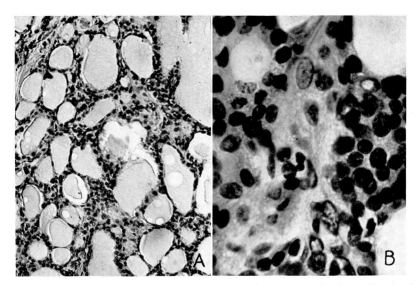

FIG. 115. Long burned-out Graves' disease which lighted up ending in cardiac death: *A*, the interacinal cells are multiplied while the acinal cells are flat and in parts defective; *B*, the cells have large deeply staining nuclei. A few cells are palely staining with large ovoid nuclei.

retreats unsung to oblivion; but the thyroid which adopts us when the thymus deserts us and which sees us to maturity, that thyroid we have cherished throughout life as something essential to our adult existence. Is this the result of good physiology or the result of Kocher jitters?

Histology. The concluding paragraph above carries enough possibilities to warrant the thyroid gland being studied anew in all its structural changes. Studied not only in terms of goiter but as an organ subject to the changes of old age, whether associated with enlargement or not.

In view of the microscopic findings of the preceding stages of goiter when cardiac failure begins there is little to offer that is new. That is to be expected. The final stage can hardly be anything else than the sum of the preceding stages. It is the sum of the preceding changes to which are added degenerative changes not present in goiters in their thyrotoxic state. It even seems likely that we are dealing entirely with ultimate results expressed in terms of degeneration and not of hyperfunction, though the former is inevitably the end stage of the latter.

Nevertheless the slide gives evidence of many of the late clinical signs. A long dormant goiter that suddenly lights up with indications of toxicity, lashing to a fatal termination an already lagging heart, is found to show

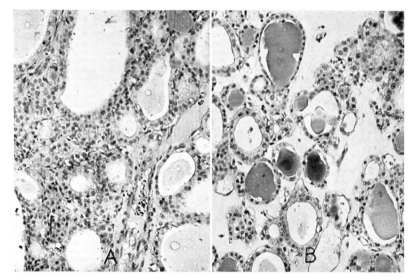

Fig. 116. Cardiotoxic goiter: *A*, the acinal cells are cuboidal with many interacinal cells; the colloid stains faintly or not at all; *B*, the same as the preceding but some of the colloid is basophilic and some of the cells show atrophy and degeneration.

hyperplasia. This is seen most exquisitely in old burned-out Basedow disease which having run a but slightly toxic course suddenly lights up and again becomes toxic (Fig. 115). But the lighting up is due to outlaw cells that lack the regularity in form or arrangement of the usually hyperplastic cells. They are interacinal in arrangement for the most part.

Others again show an awakening of the acinal epithelium, but there is evidence of a changed colloid (Fig. 116). Goiters of many years' duration, often without notable toxic symptoms—that is, they go from the nodular nontoxic directly into the cardiopathic—show little or no cellular hyperplasia, only colloid changes (Fig. 117). It would seem as though the colloid silently poisoned the heart without ever stimulating it to

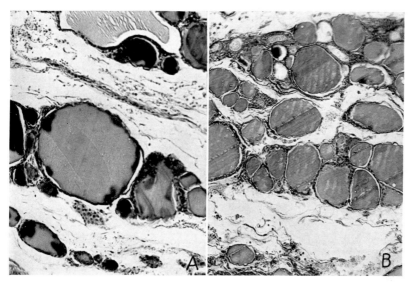

FIG. 117. Cardiotoxic goiter developed on an old colloid goiter. *A*, The epithelium is atrophied to invisibility, many acini are almost obliterated. The colloid is in part basophilic. *B*, The colloid stains deeply, the cells are atrophic and all but obscured.

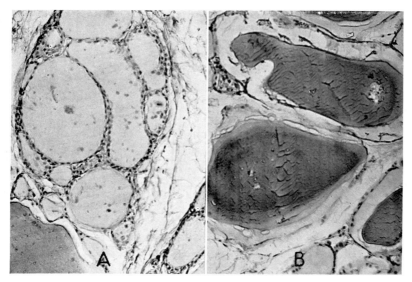

FIG. 118. Cardiotoxic colloid goiter: *A*, the acinal cells are flat, the colloid palely staining; *B*, the acinal epithelium is for the most part exfoliated. The colloid is baso-philic and retracted. Some acini are wholly devoid of epithelium, the colloid fusing with the adjacent connective tissue.

marked increased activity. This is likely to be the final stage of the fetal adenomas. The slide gives no evidence as to what it is that affects the heart. The epithelium is flat, seemingly functionally useless, surrounded by fibrous tissue which is equally inert. The cells may have actually cut loose from their base as though compressed by the basophilic colloid (Fig. 118).

The thyroid may be so changed that in some areas the nature of the tissue can hardly be recognized; isolated groups of cells being situated in areas of purposeless connective tissue (Fig. 119). Is such tissue still

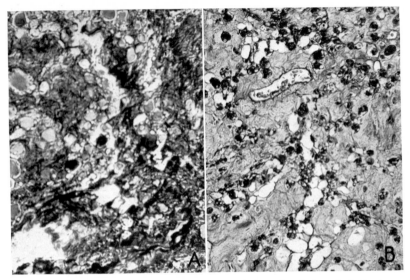

Fig. 119. Thyrocardiac goiter. The structure of the goiter is largely lost: *A*, small acini with flat cells, fibrous tissue much increased; *B*, all acini are devoid of epithelium. In some the colloid is stainless, in others deeply staining (Trichrome II stain).

producing a baneful influence? So far it seems that when such tissue is removed it allows the patient to recover all but a normal cardiac function.

The cellular degenerations are most marked in those who die in a final crescendo of wild heart, delirium and high fever. The cells apparently have started to attain a state of rejuvenation (Fig. 120). The colloid is pale, even entirely unstainable. The cells seem degenerated, beginning in the protoplasm (Fig. 121). The nuclei are disintegrated, or become contracted and stain an intense color as though giving a final wave of the hand at a cruel world.

The extreme degree of change is reached in cases where the cells are massed in acini which have lost semblance of a definite wall (Fig. 122).

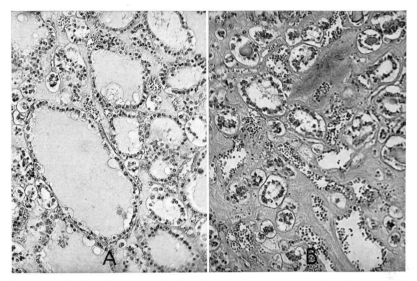

Fig. 120. Cardiotoxic goiter. Patient died unoperated on, in wild delirium. *A*, The acinal cells retain their position but show evidence of degeneration. *B*, More advanced cell destruction. Marked fibrosis. The colloid is represented only by all but stainless débris.

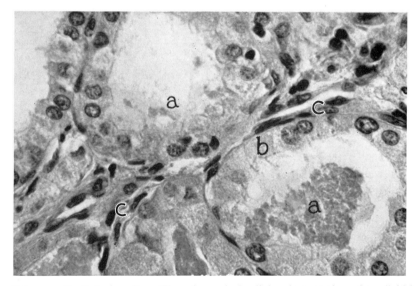

Fig. 121. Cardiotoxic goiter. There is marked cellular degeneration; the colloid is granular and stainless; *a,a*, the nuclei of some acinal cells are degenerated with others, *b*, in the process of degeneration; *c,c*, connective tissue with deeply staining nuclei.

Other areas show less marked changes but indicate that connective tissue as well as the epithelium is undergoing degeneration.

The histologic study of the heart muscle shows nothing distinctive. Those in which death follows operation usually show an increase in fibrous tissue and some brown degeneration, such as one finds in old people dying of nothing in particular. Of those who die spontaneously with a superlative of all the signs that the cardiotoxic state can inspire, some at least show an infiltration of foreign cells that are round, plasma, or what they may be. It is as though the beleaguered heart muscle had

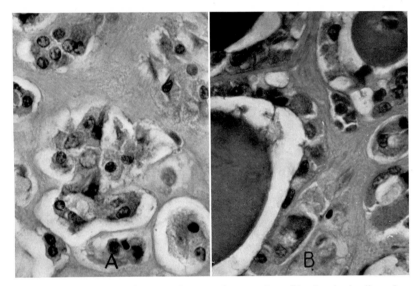

FIG. 122. Cardiotoxic goiter. *A*, Extreme degeneration of both acinal cells and connective tissue. Many of the cells are wholly disintegrated   *B*, Less marked degeneration. Basophilic colloid retained in some acini; from others it has disappeared. Acinal cells in various stages of degeneration.

short waved to the police a final protest against something that was killing it.

Unsatisfactory and inadequate as this account of the histologic changes in the cardiotoxic heart may be, it is sufficient to show that everywhere there is destruction and annihilation of everything capable of normal function. In view of these things I fail to see how any surgeon can leave part of the gland at operation and feel that he is doing his patient a service.

During the years when postoperative myxedema was a cherished fetish partial operations were logical. Now we know the premises were wrong.

Literature

Degenerative Goiter. The relation of goiters to cardiac change is such a new thing that the problem cannot even be definitely formulated. The result is that surgeons and cardiologists are still browsing in separate fields, neither quite understanding just what the other is trying to do. It is all a matter of the future. The surgeons are still too frightened to aid the cardiologists with total removal of the offending gland. Even the fundamental problem whether the cardiac disturbance is due to overstimulation of the heart by virtue of hyperplasia or as the result of the production of toxic substance the result of degenerative changes. Pathologists and physiologists have contributed chiefly nothing being content for the most part to worship at the shrines of the past.

One can do little better to list a few of the excellent papers that have been published in profusion recently. In the most of these papers the name of Blumgart stands as a guiding post. Only a few of these need be cited because these contain an abundant literature.

The October 1932 number of the *Amer. Heart Journal* is devoted to a series of most excellent papers on the thyroid heart, many of them of course too deep for the surgeon. Arn (*West. J. Surg.*, Dec. 1930, 36, 755) and Kahn (*West. J. Surg.*, May 1935, 43, 253) likewise contribute interesting papers. Last but not least the pioneering paper of Crotti (*Ohio St. Med. J.*, Feb. 15, 1912, 8, 61–66) deserves study. The paper of Davison (*South. Surg.*, June 1934, 3, 103–111) presents most clearly the clinical relations of the nodular type of goiters to cardiac conditions.

CHAPTER VIII

Atypical Toxic Goiter (Interstitial Goiter)

IN MY recent book on clinical goiter I called these "atypical toxic" goiters in preference to using the term previously employed; namely, interstitial. They are mildly toxic and they are certainly atypical when compared with other kinds of toxic goiters. If they have a distinct pathology it must be built on the presence of interstitial cells, but the colloid presents changes sometimes of dominant importance. However, any term one may apply to this condition should be regarded as a symbol rather than a designation because the chief characteristics are clinical.

My conception of the disease is based on a more or less characteristic clinical syndrome which has not been generally recognized though I believe it should be. Extensive experience in the clinic, and continued study of the slides these patients furnish, convince me that it may be tentatively accepted as a clinical entity with a basic pathology. The fact that I have been harping on this subject for more than twenty years, without exciting the least flicker of interest among my colleagues, is of itself evidence of the correctness of my observations.

It was stated in the previous chapter that certain disturbances of the thyroid gland at puberty, associated with menstrual disturbances, may be regarded as a family row among the endocrine glands which is generally adjusted after a while when each takes up its specific duty and harmony is achieved. In the type here considered a harmonious adjustment is never reached. Therefore it is something more than a disease of the thyroid gland: it is a maladjustment of several members of the endocrine system, most likely involving the pituitary as well. Because of its common association with menstrual disturbances, and the physical characteristics of the gland, it would not be unreasonable to liken it to the so-called chronic mastitis which, because of recurring irritation from the menstrual function, finally undergoes a certain permanent change. However, in view of some changes continually discerned in the thyroid gland it is more likely that the primary disturbance is to be found here and that the ovarian disturbance is secondary to it. Broadly speaking, the microscopic findings suggest a relationship to the infantile gland which warrants the tentative conclusion that the gland never has reached an adult state and that it is this developmental frustration which causes the general disturbance. There are conjoint regressive changes in the colloid,

148

associated with the interstitial cells, and are often present in glands in which the interstitial cells are absent. There is still a third type occasionally observed; namely, that in which many lymphoid nodules are present. This kind is more or less suffused. Generally speaking, the less one understands a disease the more necessary is an elaborate classification. It serves to keep in mind certain factors when one is studying a concrete case that does not fit into any of the classes.

Every other therapeutic measure having failed to bring relief to these patients, I began some six years ago to do complete thyroidectomies in selected cases. The idea was to determine the dominant factor in the symptom complex. The result has been satisfactory to both patient and surgeon. Obviously any procedure that appears as radical as complete thyroidectomy does to most surgeons demands a careful presentation of facts relative to the postoperative course and clinical results. In comparison the microscopic study is of secondary importance.

The study therefore is a complicated one since the basis must, for the present, be clinical. Even the clinical recognition may be difficult, for the nervousness manifested may be closely simulated by diseases of the nervous system or by purely functional conditions in no wise related to the thyroid disease. However, the anatomic findings are such that they offer sufficient objective evidence to aid in reaching clinical conclusions. That is to say, if the anatomic changes detailed below are absent, one can be certain that he has operated on a neurotic, anticipating by some months what the after-course will reveal. On the other hand, if the histologic changes are present one can confidently predict satisfactory results.

The problem, therefore, divides itself into two parts: the preoperative clinical study on which we base an opinion as to what is wrong, and the anatomic study of the tissues removed which confirms or confutes that opinion. Clinically three groups may be recognized. There is the high type of individual who is usually of good physique but always at high tension, and tormented by nervousness of which she complains though there is no outward manifestation of it. The constitutionally substandard, which is the classical type, gives evidence of weakness, fatigability, a somewhat rapid pulse, suffers sleeplessness and a varying degree of loss in weight. The third type, dominatingly dysmenorrhoeic, may show evidence of an associated hypo state and sometimes of a pituitary complication.

Anatomically there are likewise three types. The first shows a gland that is cellularly a simple colloid goiter but one with pronounced tinctorial changes in the colloid and with or without associated interstitial cells. The second presents clusters of cells in the interacinal cells and more or less change in the colloid. This is the common type which forms the basis of this chapter. The third type may present either of the above or a combination of both, with a conspicuously large number of lymph follicles scattered throughout the gland.

Pathogenesis. Before attempting to particularize, I wish first to present a general picture of the disease seen in the clinic. I quote a paragraph from my clinical goiter book: "An atypical toxic goiter is a symptom-complex characterized by a small, uniform, firm elastic goiter, a general nervous irritability, a moderately rapid pulse, usually a slight loss in weight and, in most cases, an associated menstrual disturbance; all this embodied in a constitution that has never been quite up to par. These patients are thin, small-boned, delicate in looks, and retiring in demeanor. They are withal intellectual, high minded, and are prone to haunt the seats of learning. Impressive is the unchangeable chronicity, the symptoms continuing with little or no change either in the goiter or in the associated symptoms for many years. The whole picture impresses one as being something apart from the usual goiter with its tendency to progress from one stage to another. Because of the associated menstrual disturbances, which indicate pituitary and ovarian unbalance, a polyglandular disease is suggested rather than a pure disturbance of the thyroid gland."

Members of the first group just mentioned present a variation from the above in that they are not particularly inferior constitutionally though they are not robust. They are nervous, but it is an unvarying nervousness which drives them constantly to overtax their strength and impels a perennial recourse to tonics and sedatives. This type, it may be mentioned in advance, is characterized by colloid changes parallel with those discussed in the chapter on nontoxic nodular except that this disease is nonprogressive, and there is no new formation of acini, hence no formation of nodules.

In the second group above noted the patients seem to be constitutionally marked from the beginning. They are slender, illy nourished; they lack vitality and tend to intellectual habits. They usually begin to menstruate late and it is painful from the start. The constitution remains delicate, they are easily exhausted. The pulse rate is increased but the metabolism is not. At intervals they may lose a few pounds in weight, but though small such losses vitally affect these delicate constitutions. In general the picture suggests what neurologists, when pressed for a diagnosis, have called neurovascular neurasthenia.

The essential feature of the disease, it cannot be repeated too often, is the unvarying chronicity. It is this chronicity which warrants one in regarding it as a thyroid state rather than a thyroid disease, as a mal-development rather than a regression from what was once normal. To appreciate this unvarying state one should for a time observe these patients on sedative medication in order to separate the inherent nervous element which is often the result of a faulty environment; this may be necessary before a definite diagnosis can be made, for neurotics some-times have goiters.

Those patients who marry usually have a child or two, and then all the ills listed above are aggravated and they sink into complaining in-validism. To the plight imposed by their disease are added the disap-pointments of domestic life which engenders a resentful, self-pitying state that makes the prognosis much more unfavorable than in the case of the unwed individual who has escaped the joys of marital discord with their sinister mental influences. One may change the physical state but not the mental. These patients are not categorically to be refused operation, but the added factors must be weighed in estimating the postoperative prognosis. The state of the pelvis and the social habits of the conjugal pair must be taken into account. Often such patients are on the threshold of the divorce court, for a total 'ectomy is no substitute for a judge and a pair of scissors.

The disease seems to be rare in males. The few on whom I have tried total 'ectomies were not so satisfactory as in the case of women. One, at first apparently a failure, responded satisfactorily with the use of pituitary extract. Another diagnosed in the clinic a sexual neurasthenic and apparently a cerebral hermaphrodite, ended in eloquent failure, or so it seemed; but after pouring forth reams of lamentations for a year he finally concluded that he felt quite well. I also tried the operation on a neurotic woman who was mad at her husband. It did no good; it must be the adrenals.

The third, the pituitary type, is remarkable chiefly for the excessive development of hair, even to a point suggestive of a male type. There have been too few to warrant even tentative conclusions. The nervous state in the few operated on seemed to improve but the hair development seemed to increase.

It is a matter of historical interest to note that the ovarian pains associated with this type of goiter present the picture which for many years led to the diagnosis of chronic appendicitis and cystic ovaries. Now, since we know that chronic appendicitis occurs only in dodo birds, and that cystic ovaries are only ova which got tired waiting, this symptom complex no longer incites needless operations.

The study of the after-course following a total thyroidectomy is of the greatest interest since the operation seems to violate our most cherished physiological notion of the thyroid gland; to wit, that the entire gland cannot be removed without producing the dire results described by Kocher. After a careful reading of Kocher's article I discovered that in none of the cases in which he did the total operation in adults did his cachexia thyreopriva result. This discovery made me much less hesitant in doing complete thyroidectomy. Being sensible of a considerable responsibility for inaugurating such a radical therapeutic measure, because many surgeons are still horrified at the very thought of so extreme a procedure, I shall discuss the final results. This is important also from a theoretical viewpoint. Since some of these cases at least appear to involve several of the endocrine glands, what happens when one link of the chain is removed may throw light on the function of the others. It can be stated most emphatically that cachexia thyreopriva did not occur in my cases any more than it did in Kocher's (See lit., chapter on myxedema). Several did show temporary clinical myxedema but recovered on the use of thyroid extract for a few months. None has required the extract permanently. The youngest operated on was 19 years of age. No myxedema resulted and she is one of my most brilliant results, having been relieved of a very severe dysmenorrhea and the general physical disturbance. The best results, on the whole, have been obtained in cases who were between 30 and 40 years of age at the time of operation. These are less likely to be disturbed by fleeting nervous states of anticipation, or realization. In some of the patients there was a considerable gain in weight with puffiness of the face for a few months after operation. Some of these took small doses of thyroid extract for a few months, allegedly with benefit. Other patients with similar disturbances did as well on the Syrup of the Iodide of Iron, and some equally well on no medication at all. For a year there has been no evidence of thyroid deficiency. On the whole the minimum age for operation is now 25 years, though quite a number of very satisfactory results were obtained in patients in the early twenties.

The final results depend much on the type of patient. Nervous symptoms independent of goiter and commonly seen in neurotic patients remain of course. These are often difficult to determine before operation and only reach full tongue, as the fox hunters say, after the operation. It is the easily exhausted type, those doing their honest best in some intellectual pursuit and who sleep poorly and are in a tense but ambiguously described nervous state, that most completely recover after operation. However, there are limits to what even a normal constitution can bear. Many of these patients, finding their capacity for work increased, quickly extend their labors and use up the added energy. A study of the patient's environment after operation is important. For an unhappy home life may retard or even prevent recovery; the operation is in no wise a substitute for the divorce court.

How shall we co-ordinate observations made after total thyroidectomy with the accepted teachings of physiology? I make no such attempt—

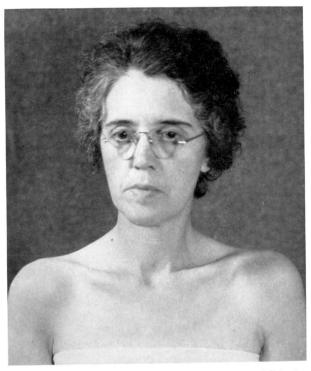

FIG. 123. Slight tenseness of the sternomastoid muscle with a visible thyroid enlargement. Typical slender intellectual type.

that is the business of the physiologists. Our duty ends with the recording of the facts. However, it would seem, even to a surgeon, that perhaps when once we have grown up the thyroid gland is not as essential to our welfare as we have been led to believe. We need proof that, having attained adult development, the thyroid gland is of any use to us. This theme is more fully discussed in the chapter on morphology.

If anybody cares, it can be stated that totally 'ectomized patients have on the average a basal rate of minus 10 to 15, about, in fact, what they had before operation and what our bright husky pupil nurses have.

Dependence on the basal machine has done about as much to obfuscate us as did the misreading of Kocher's paper, published more than half a century ago.

Pathology. Pathologists are prone to regard with disdain the surgeon's presentation of the patient's general appearance as an integral part of the study of the pathology of a disease, just as we do when

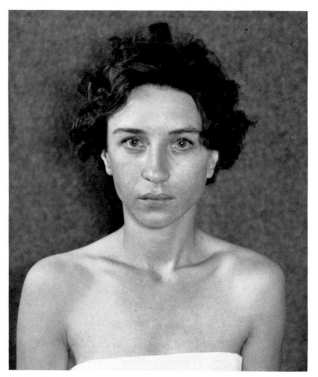

Fig. 124. Slight tenseness of the sternomastoid muscle without visible thyroid enlargement.

the laboratory report talks of chromosomes in an obviously malignant tumor.

The study of the general appearance in this type of goiter is important because the peculiar kind of nervousness from which these patients suffer is inarticulate and one must divine it by the appearance as noted in the clinic.

In the higher types which are fully developed physically the appearance is that of quiet dignity, and only the tenseness of the neck muscles bespeaks a nervous tension (Fig. 123). The typical case presents a general tenseness of the whole body, most pronounced in the sterno-mastoids (Fig. 124). The more extreme cases, marked by lack of physical development, show the tenseness in a more extreme degree (Fig. 125). Those associated with pituitary disturbances may be overweight and may present signs of submyxedema (Fig. 126).

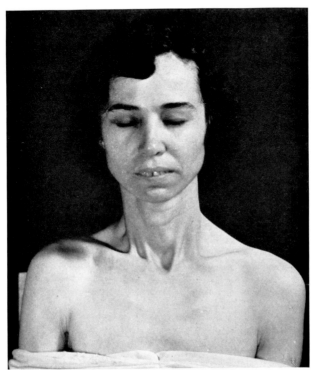

Fɪɢ 125. Very obvious tension of the sternomastoid muscles and a visible thyroid enlargement.

The study of the pathologic anatomy must begin in the clinic. Often the size and form of the thyroid enlargement becomes apparent when the patient elevates her chin (Fig. 127). The feel of the thyroid gland is a most constant part of the picture. It is slightly and uniformly enlarged, from two to four times the normal size in most cases. More conspicuous than the enlargement is the increased density. It differs in this respect from the small goiters of adolescence, being firmer, but less firm than distinctly toxic goiters. In some cases it is a question whether one would recognize any thyroid gland at all, so slight is it, were it not for the associated clinical conditions which lead to careful search for glandular enlargement. The thyroids are not fixed to the surrounding structures, nor do they have the sensitiveness of the more active glands of acutely toxic goiters. The patient may complain of sensitiveness to pressure, however. This very sign should suggest pure nervousness and put the surgeon on his guard.

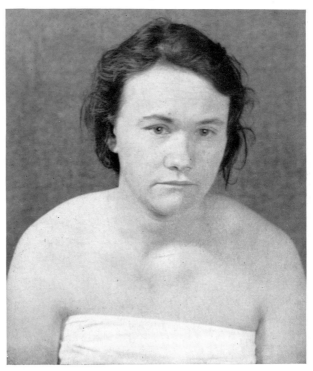

FIG. 126. Submyxedematoid type of interstitial goiter. Age 23 at time of operation. Required thyroid extract for some months after operation. Did not require it for two years but recently showed some evidence for its need.

The peculiarities of the pathologic anatomy become apparent during the operation. The glands do not pop out when the vessels are severed, as do the simple colloid, nor is the tissue friable as in very toxic goiters. The capsule is in a measure attached to the environment, hence when the gland is removed it presents a woolly specimen despite the most careful technic (*A*, Fig. 128). The gland may show definite bosselations (*A*, Fig. 129).

The external form is that of the normal gland, save that it is uniformly larger. The firmer consistency after removal, as in the clinic, is the chief gross characteristic.

The cross-section is notable. The fibrous bands are as prominent as in the infant gland, and divide the field into compartments (*B*, Fig. 128). This confirms the general impression that the gland, like the patient, has never fully grown up. For it is an undeveloped infantile gland. The

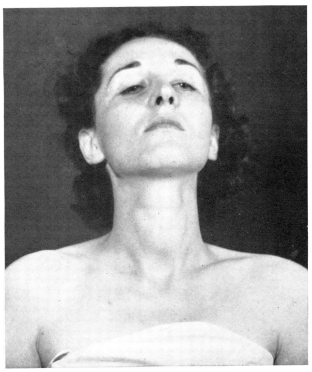

FIG. 127. Uniform interstitial goiter. The size and outline of the thyroid gland is easily made out. The size, general outline of the gland and its position in the neck is very characteristic.

fibrous septa may be much thickened and areas of fibrous tissue are sometimes seen (*B*, Fig. 129). The gland may, on the whole, have the gross appearance of a senile gland (Fig. 130), being elastic and but little enlarged. This type of gland is most commonly seen in older patients. These small hard glands remind me in physical characters and microscopic structure of incipient Hashimoto goiters. Small fetal adenomas are commonly surprise findings of the cross-section (Fig. 129). These have no part in the general picture of the disease.

Small fibrous areas are sometimes observed in these goiters (Fig. 131), with lobulations not so definitely fibrous. These areas are associated with lymphatic infiltration which are really localized Hashimoto changes. They differ from those in which the lymph follicles appear as a congenital state.

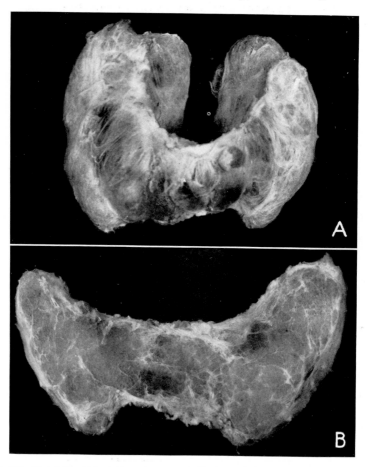

Fig. 128. Total thyroidectomy. Age 23. *A*, Surface of the gland showing the fibrous irregular capsule. The gland nearly surrounded the trachea. *B*, Cut surface showing the fibrous septa and the obviously thickened capsule.

Not the least interesting part of this study is the course after total thyroidectomy. The effect on nutrition and digestion is important in connection with the possible etiology of gastric ulcer. The stomach complaints disappear in most cases. Such patients invariably ceased to call for their bromides after operation. Some required thyroid extract for a period of months; a few took it at intervals for several years. Occasionally there is little or no improvement and the explanation of such cases is found in a study of the slide—one has simply removed a normal gland.

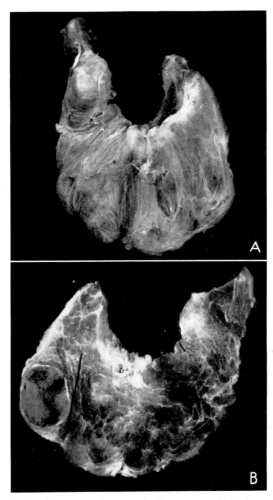

FIG. 129. Total thyroidectomy. Age 33. *A*, The upper pole is elongated and the surface of the gland is somewhat bosselated. *B*, The cross-section shows extensive fibrous tissue septa and incidentally on the left a fetal adenoma.

A renewed study of the clinical history of these cases often reveals factors mentioned above, chiefly domestic. One must not become discouraged too soon. If the slide shows the characteristic changes, described below, improvement will come though its appearance may be delayed a year or more. This fact would indicate that the changes are specific.

The effect on the preoperative dysmenorrhea is variable. The general tendency is toward gradual improvement, and the younger the patient the more likely is this to hold.

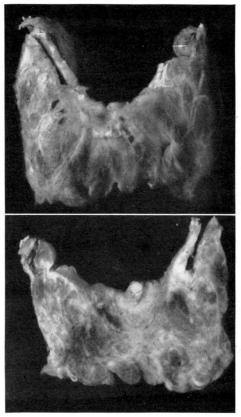

FIG. 130. Total thyroidectomy. F., age 43. The gland was but little enlarged but was markedly fibrous. The clinical results were such that the patient asked why the operation had not been done long before.

I want again to present the patient who required thyroid extract after operation (Fig. 126). As previously stated she was of the submyx-edematoid type before operation, as is obvious from the features. There is a marked contrast with the previous patients shown. In retrospect it is clear that she belongs in Chapter XI.

Histology. The record of the microscopic study of this disease is simply a record of the findings of the tissue removed by total thyroidectomy. The basis was clinical. However, two definite changes have been constantly present, collections of cells lying in the spaces between the acini, and the tinctorial changes in the colloid.

A third factor is the presence of islands of cells in the spaces between the acini above mentioned.

The typical picture is one in which the cells of the larger acini are flat or low cuboid with the angles between the several alveoli filled with cells (Fig. 132). The general picture is that of the goiter of a child which

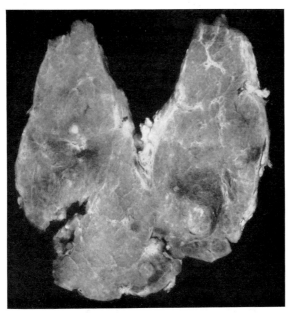

FIG. 131. Total 'ectomy in a patient aged 44 years. She was treated for nervousness for 21 years before operation was undertaken. There is a general lobular fibrosis with definitely sclerotic areas.

normally presents these islands of cells lying between the acini containing colloid. The attempt to explain these cell groups as prolongations from the tips of converging acini is as futile as it is unnecessary. They are normal in childhood and the simplest explanation is that they are a persistence of these cells. This is particularly logical since there is commonly associated an obvious lack of physical development. This view is supported by the presence of areas resembling the embryonal structure of fetal adenomas (Fig. 133).

Some areas show acini with tall epithelium (Fig. 134). These cases exhibit evidence of hypersecretion. They also present clinical pictures

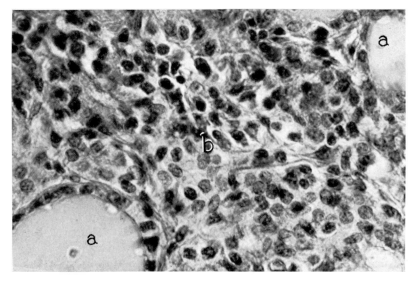

Fig. 132. Interstitial cells lying between several typical acini: *a,a,* acini relatively normal; *b,* interstitial cells are of the same size and stain identically with those lining the acini. Nowhere is there evidence of a lumen nor is there demonstrable any connection with adjacent acini. (×450).

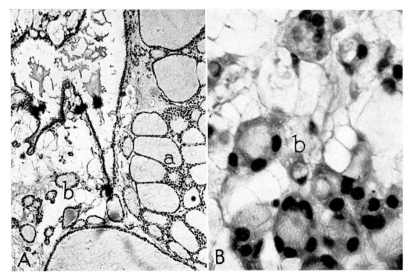

Fig. 133. Fetal rest in an interstitial goiter: *A,* an area of fetal tissue, *a,* is separated from the normal gland which made up the greater part of the goiter, *b; B,* the acini are small, defectively lined and the colloid negligible; the connective tissue is illy formed.

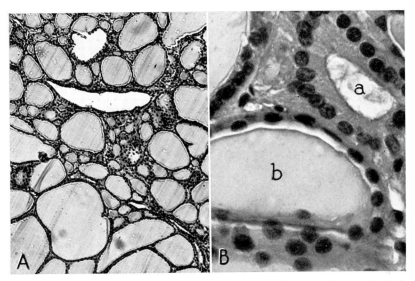

FIG. 134. Interstitial goiter: *A*, large acini lined with flat epithelium with limited interstitial small acini, some nuclei without lumina; *B*, *a*, small acinus with tall epithelium and imperfect colloid; *b*, old acinus with flat epithelium and homogeneous basophilic colloid.

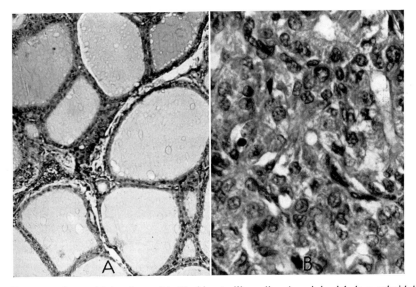

FIG. 135. Interstitial goiter with Hashimoto-like cells: *A*, acini with low cuboidal cells and a uniform palely staining colloid; *B*, cells with large vesicular nuclei with abundant protoplasm more or less suffused with adjacent cells. Some nuclei are degenerated.

of a combination of interstitial goiter with a hyperplastic one. These are most likely to be observed in the clinical group I mentioned above.

In some cases the cells are suffused and the protoplasm stains deeply with eosin (Fig. 135). They are identical in appearance with the acini in Hashimoto's disease. Such pictures as this are seen most commonly in submyxedematoid states.

Of equal interest are the areas in which the acini are lined with deeply

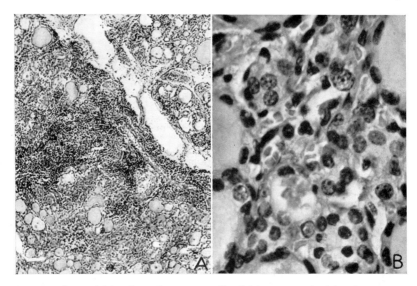

Fig. 136. Interstitial goiter: *A*, many small acini interspersed with acinal cells and lymphocytes; *B*, the acinal cells are large with granular nuclei, irregularly arranged, and intermingled cells with deeply staining nuclei, probably lymphocytes.

staining cells quite like those in the interstitial tissue. In some of the acini the epithelium is defective (Fig. 136).

The tinctorial changes in the colloid are particularly noteworthy. Even in cases in which the interstitial cells are not conspicuous these colloid changes are found. They may therefore be regarded as the most constant feature. Many show basophilic changes with hematoxylin-eosin, particularly in the colloid in the larger acini (Fig. 137). When no change is shown in the hematoxylin-eosin slides it is shown in the more sensitive dyes, such as a methylene blue slide (Fig. 138). This indicates an inactive colloid which is in harmony with the flat epithelium. It is of interest to note, though the significance is unknown, that the colloid retracts with bichromate hardening while normal colloid does not.

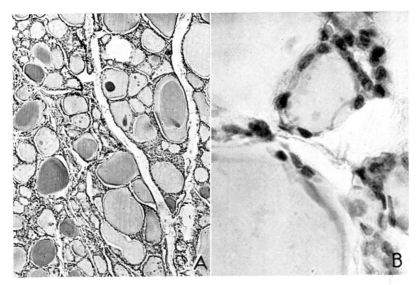

FIG. 137. Basophilic changes in the colloid and defective epithelium in some of the acini. *A*, The colloid in the various acini shows a varying degree of stainability by hematoxylin. *B*, Acini have a defective cell lining, particularly the large one.

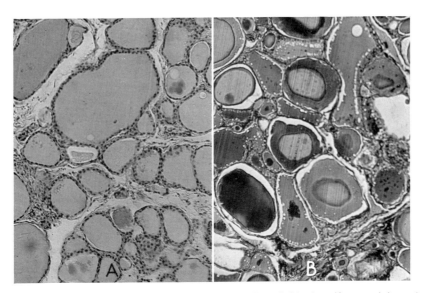

FIG. 138. Interstitial goiter showing changes in the colloid: *A*, uniform staining colloid with hematoxylin-eosin; *B*, variable staining colloid with Mallory's methylene blue. The changes are usually most marked in the periphery in the beginning. ($\times$110)

Whatever of value this pathologic study may have, the fact remains that these patients do not become myxedemic; and, to say the least, they are clinically vastly benefited.

Literature

Interstitial. This ill defined chapter possesses little literature: Goetsch (*Endocrinology*, 1920, 4, 389) and Hertzler (Diseases of the Thyroid Gland, Mosby, St. Louis, 1922; *J. Missouri M. A.*, 1922, 19, 207). The former dropped the subject after the single paper but the latter has persisted to grope more or less in the dark trying to fit a definite clinical picture with an indefinite anatomic finding. Just recently Davison (Chronic Hyperthyroidism With a Persistently Low Basal Metabolism Rate, *J. M. A. Georgia*, July 1936, vol. xxv, No. 7) has hit on a nomenclature which is at once comprehensive and prejudices nothing, to wit, "chronic toxic goiter." From the pathologic side Hertzler (*Am. J. Surg.*, March 1934, 23, 556–558) by total thyroidectomies has secured satisfying clinical improvement by the total removal of the gland providing this material for anatomic study. From another side Blumgart's welcome support by doing total 'ectomies for cardiac conditions has helped much in alleviating the fright the profession has so long entertained at the very thought of removing too much of the thyroid gland. The total result is that we are now in a position to study this pathologic state in the clinic by radical operation and in consequence in the laboratory by virtue of the material so obtained.

CHAPTER IX

Toxic Diffuse Goiter

(*Exophthalmic Goiter, Graves' Disease, Basedow's Disease*)

THE array of synonyms given in the caption of this chapter might well have been extended to thirty or more. While the term "toxic diffuse" by no means covers the field completely, because not all are diffuse, it is on the whole satisfactory in the clinic as well as the laboratory. Basedow's disease is synonymous with exophthalmic goiter, whereas Graves' disease covers all types of goiter, including the nodular which are or become acutely toxic. Therefore, there is something more than national pride which should govern the use of these eponyms, if one must use them—they are not synonyms.

One may define diffuse toxic goiter as that type of thyroid disease in which, as the result of unknown factors, hyperplasia of the epithelial cells takes place and results in acute toxic symptoms, consisting of rapid pulse, loss of weight, increased capillary circulation, tremor, and in some cases, protrusion of the eyeballs. Because of its acute onset and common occurrence in young patients the outline of the gland as seen in the clinic is usually uniform.

When it occurs later in life and is sometimes implanted on old nontoxic or toxic nodular goiters it is called secondary toxic. This is proper enough if we remember that the hyperactivity is due to epithelial hyperplasia as distinguished from the degenerative form. These secondary toxic goiters are usually less acute in onset and less typical than those that develop in earlier life. In general, one may say that it is easy to understand why this is so because in young persons the epithelium is more labile and responds more promptly and more extensively to stimuli than in the old gland which has already undergone some changes incident to advanced years. Certain it is that the older the person the less likely is acute goiter to develop in typical form.

Whether the diffuse acute goiter develops on a goitrous gland or on one previously normal has been much discussed. In many patients I have had the chance to observe a simple diffuse nontoxic goiter for a considerable time, for several years in a few cases, before the more or less sudden advent of acute toxic signs. One knows certainly therefore that

167

in some cases this disease may develop on the base of the diffuse nontoxic goiter. In other cases one does not know whether or not a nontoxic goiter existed before the advent of toxic signs. The patient presents herself with a well developed case, not having had occasion previously to undergo a physical examination. In some cases not previously examined there is pathologic evidence of a pretoxic goiter, notably large distended acini with flat epithelium interspersed with the hyperplasia which characterizes this disease. In cases when there are no distended acini, it seems fair to assume that there was no preceding enlargement—at least one has a right to assume that there was. Of course in cases in which a colloid nontoxic goiter has long preceded the acute disease, the answer to the question as to which belongs to the old and which to the new becomes perfectly obvious in the laboratory. The new hyperplasia is as conspicuous as a new sprout on an old all but dead stump of a tree. True exophthalmic goiter implanted on an old colloid goiter is rare. Usually the toxic manifestations stop far short of this, as was noted in the chapter on the nodular toxic.

In general one may distinguish two types of toxic diffuse goiter, those with and those without eye signs. The division is not sharp, however, for a diffuse toxic goiter may exist for a time without eye signs, and then present protrusion of the eyeballs. In days gone by, when all goiters were treated by nonoperative measures, it was not unusual to observe this transition. There would be a gradual increase in degree of toxicity without eye signs, followed within weeks, or even days, by pronounced eye signs. These observations are of interest because they show the essential affinity of the two groups, those with eye signs and those without. The appearance of the eye signs may be regarded as the final step in completing the set-up. Nowadays one sees this transition less often because removal of the gland is undertaken, and properly so, in the earlier stages.

Usually when a goiter that is very acutely toxic is implanted on a bosselated nontoxic colloid goiter the signs are less pronounced. The capillary manifestations and tremor in particular are less conspicuous and even though the general symptoms all approach a similar intense degree, eye signs rarely develop. Apparently the pre-existing goiter so affects the acinal epithelium that the peculiar hyperplasia characteristic of the exophthalmic type, or degree, cannot develop. There is therefore a fundamental difference between the diffuse toxic as we see it in young persons and that which develops on an old colloid goiter. The difference fundamentally concerns the individual acini.

It is worthy of note that these secondary toxic goiters, even though the symptoms are less pronounced, are more serious than the truer classical type because the old colloid goiter has already damaged the heart, and the acute hyperplasia brings disaster. This fact is more impressive in the clinic, particularly postoperatively, than in the laboratory.

Much needless confusion has been caused in the study of the pathology of acute toxic goiter chiefly because of too cursory examination of the tissue removed at operation. It is not unusual to find different parts of a goiter unequally affected. Affected areas frequently are interspersed in simple colloid goiter, as was noted in the chapter on goiters in children. Sometimes one entire lobe is affected while the entire other lobe remains simple colloid. If the typical pathologic changes of acute toxic goiter are not found in the first block of tissue examined, further search is necessary. After repeated examinations never once in my experience have I failed to find the characteristic changes. If there are eye signs there is papillary hyperplasia in the gland; conversely, if there is papillary hypertrophy in the gland one may be sure that the patient had eye signs. There is no more constant relationship between the pathologic and the clinical in all surgical pathology.

In some cases the greater part of the gland may show simple colloid goiter—the younger the patient, the more likely is this to be the case— or small nonpapillated acini though some regions will show the papillations. The failure to recognize this fact has led to the publication of pictures of slides taken from exophthalmic goiters which showed simple smooth balloon-like acini. Certainly, one may admit that such material was removed from a patient who had exophthalmic goiter, but one might as well excise a block from a normal area of a breast, in a case of mammary carcinoma, and then categorically deny the specificity of epithelial proliferation in cancer of the breast. The picture is not overdrawn.

Let it be added here that there is more to the histology of the thyroid gland in toxic goiters than is expressed by mere increase in the acinal epithelium. If the epithelial proliferation in a toxic goiter seems to be out of line with the kind and degree of symptoms, one will find other changes in some areas, notably a very thin nonstainable colloid, or it may be granular and irregularly staining. This state is commonly found in the hyperacute cases which end in spontaneous death. The statement is repeatedly made that the acini are empty of colloid. By this is meant that it does not accept any dye the observer may have used. To say there is nothing in them may be an assumption. Certainly the failure to demonstrate the colloid by employing the usual laboratory stains is no evidence of its absence. However, in hyperacute cases the acini may contain only a clump of illy staining colloid, the remainder of the space showing nothing at all. In this the acinal cells are in such a state of hyperplasia that an empty lumen is maintained like the arch of a bridge. Also small acini may have no lumina. Such obviously contain no colloid. That large, thin-walled acini should remain distended though empty is just plain defiance of the ordinary laws of physics. It should be remembered that there is a difference between absence and failure to demonstrate. Poor fishermen also sometimes fail to make this distinction.

The clinical judgment of surgeons, I regret to admit, is not infallible, and when the clinical diagnosis and the pathologic structure disagree the lamentable fact had best be recognized that the surgeon was wrong. Herein lies, I may say in passing, the great advantage to the surgeon of studying his own material: it is much less of a jolt to the ego to discover one's error, say in the still hours of the night, than to have them emblazoned on the hospital chart by the pathologist.

Pathogenesis. What starts off previously normal or colloid glands, as the case may be, on their course of wild proliferation and increased secretion is not known. Speculations as to the possibilities are the business of pathologists. The student of surgical pathology will do well to stick to demonstrable facts. To him the influence of the sympathetic, or even the parasympathetic nervous system, on the production of toxic goiter can find little place, attractive as the theory may be to the poetically minded.

Severe nervous shock is believed by some to have an etiologic influence. Seldom is the previous state of the thyroid gland known, hence the time when symptoms begin cannot be determined. Attorneys for the plaintiff often desire the surgeon to recall such cases. Admittedly nervous trauma may aggravate a pre-existing case, but that any nervous shock may produce such a state in a previously normal gland has, so far as I know, not been demonstrated.

Much speculation has been indulged in as to the nature of the disease; whether it be primarily a thyroid disease or a nervous affection. Surgeons are prone to believe that disappearance of symptoms after the goiter is removed constitutes proof that it is wholly a disease of the thyroid gland. If a boy makes a lot of racket with a drum and someone destroys the drum, the noise ceases. Since there is no other way of stopping that noise, it makes little difference if the boy or the drum arrived first. Mother knows that breaking the drum is as effective as killing the boy.

Yet at the same time, as has been pointed out by a number of writers, the resemblance of exophthalmic goiter symptoms to fright is striking. That the adrenals are stimulated by nervous excitement which in turn stimulates the thyroid to hyperplasia is an attractive theory. A barrel, to one who has lost all of his clothes, may serve a useful purpose, yet there are arguments against its use as a permanent garb.

In most cases the onset of toxicity is relatively rapid, and is accompanied by nervousness, general weakness, particularly of the legs, sleeplessness, tachycardia and rapid loss of weight. The effect is constitutional but that does not make it a constitutional disease. In tetanus the effects are widespread but the lesion is local. The general constitutional conditions may continue as such, or the eye signs may develop within a few months, although they may be delayed for years—in one of my cases they failed to appear for eight years. Careful study of the glands removed at operation leaves no doubt but that the signs and the anatomic changes click perfectly and so far as the surgeon is concerned it is a local disease, something that it is within his power to remove. In our present blissful ignorance it is a surgical disease.

One of the characteristic features of the disease is that after attaining a certain degree of intensity which it maintains for a time, it then regresses to relative quiescence. Whosoever is treating the patient when this occurs secures the credit for the improvement. This fact gives the naturopath, no matter what the subvariety, his great opportunity. One speaks in such cases of the goiter having "burned out" and, in truth, the phrase is justified in many cases. There is in time a regression of the hyperplasia and the patient achieves a state of comparative well being which may endure for many years.

How long it takes for organic changes to occur is all very ambiguous. One takes out one lobe and the patient improves greatly in the succeeding three months or even three years; and then one removes the other lobe, and lo—the structure of the epithelium is the same in the two lobes! Improvement must be looked for in the colloid, not the epithelium. The regression of toxic symptoms does not spell the spontaneous cure of the disease in any case. Even when regression is permanent it is due to a degeneration of the colloid as well as of the epithelium which results in a state that affects the heart exactly like the late stages of a colloid goiter. The usual end of both is death by heart failure.

These observations are of fundamental importance. Whether the disease be constitutional or local only the removal of the goiter secures the patient against further disaster. I have followed the spontaneous "cures" for thirty years only to see them die of goiter heart.

The onset of exophthalmic goiter may be very acute, reaching its height in a few days or weeks and perhaps ending fatally in a few weeks; but it is a very rare occurrence when a case goes on to spontaneous death, even though the symptoms are so severe as to reach delirium and high fever. Diarrhea is not rare in several cases and is without special significance, but vomiting and jaundice usually presage a fatal termination. One may think of the diarrhea as a nervous manifestation but a degenerated liver is inexplicable unless other factors are considered.

Though the heart beats very rapidly, even to the limits of computability, cardiac failure is not common in acute toxic goiters and this

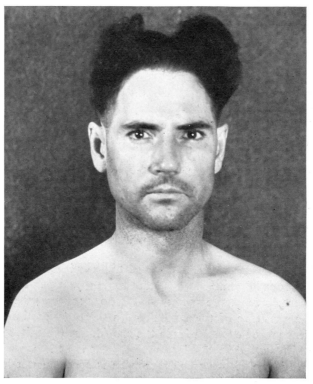

Fig. 139. Early eye signs of exophthalmic goiter. The fixed gaze was the only sign present.

indicates that the heart is merely stimulated and not diseased. It is only when the heart has been weakened by long continuance of the goiter that there is actual cardiac involvement. When this occurs the gland shows evidence of degeneration, just as in old colloid goiters.

One sign is peculiarly significant: if in the height of the illness the goiter suddenly becomes smaller even to the disappearing point, the fatal end is usually not far away. These are cases in which the colloid is granular or stains faintly or not at all. This suggests a sudden throwing into the circulation of the acinal contents, but it is more, as is evidenced by the associated changes in the structure of the acinal cells.

There is no disease about which so much can be learned by a careful study of the goiter. In days gone by when all we did was to watch the patient get worse, it was easy to follow the gradual development of the symptoms. The increased nervousness, loss of weight, the cutaneous

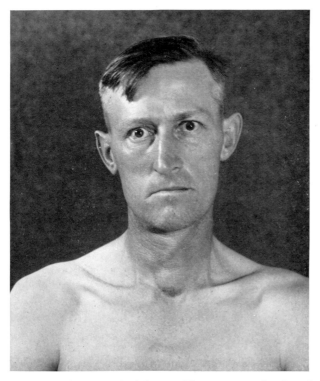

FIG. 140. Widening of the palpebral fissure. There was associated marked delay of winking.

manifestations and the tremor developed week by week, or month by month. The development of the eye signs especially is impressive and can be appreciated only by observation. The fixed gaze comes first (Fig. 139). Other signs may be absent; the widened palpebral fissure comes next, which, with the associated delayed winking, presents the first positive sign (Fig. 140).

The protrusion of the eyeball varies much in extent and in time of onset. The impressiveness of the prominence varies in the different physical types (Fig. 141). There is no accurate means of measuring the degree of protrusion; one can only estimate it by observing the patient from time to time. Unilateral exophthalmos is sometimes observed but unequal development is more common.

It is interesting sometimes to observe that the first days after operation the prominence may increase only to regress soon after. The degree of recovery after thyroidectomy is dependent on the duration of the disease. If of only short duration all but complete recovery may be ex-

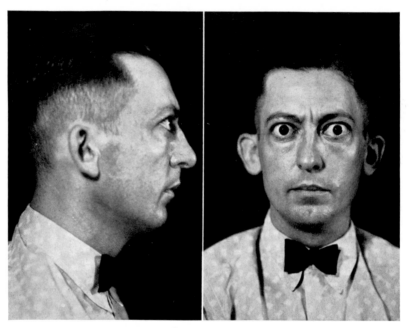

FIG. 141. Exophthalmic goiter, side and front view, showing degree of protrusion.

pected. Regression is prompt and is usually notable in a few months (Fig. 142). Occasionally one eye regresses more rapidly or more completely than the other.

On the other hand, with patients who go unoperated on, even though the general symptoms regress, the eye signs remain but little changed (Fig. 143).

Pathology. In the clinic, if the case is acute, inspection tells the whole story. The usually obvious thyroid enlargement, the pulsating vessels of the neck, the active capillary circulation, the tremor, even the loss in weight, may be obvious on examination. If eye signs are added, the frightened expression which is due to the retracted lids and the lessened rate of winking, completes the picture.

Palpation discovers the gland to be uniformly enlarged, hard; the surface is finely granular and often sensitive to the touch, though this may be expressive of apprehension rather than actual pain. Usually the enlargement is not very great; it may be very small and lie so low that it is difficult, even impossible, to feel. If preceded by a simple colloid, the gland may be large and relatively soft, particularly in young persons.

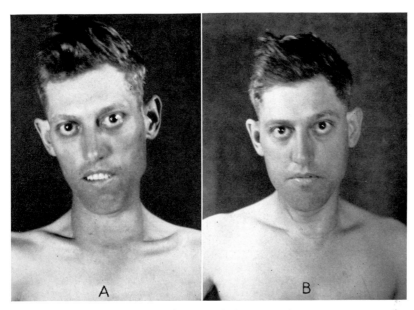

FIG. 142. Pronounced exophthalmos: *A*, before operation; *B*, two months after operation.

In the clinic this type of goiter is manifest by a uniform hard gland which is sometimes sensitive to pressure and may be more or less fixed to the adjacent structures. These suggest some reactive changes on the surface of the gland, indicating the formation of an irritating exudate in the connective tissue about the acini and reaching to and beyond the capsule. This is an expression of increased vascularity and the exudation of a tissue irritant that is local in effect. Its recognition is of importance to the operating surgeon in estimating the risk and in selecting the best time for the removal of the goiter. A gland fixed by the reaction of the capsule presages a difficult operation and represents a risk that can be avoided. It is necessary that the gland as well as the patient should be ready when the operation is undertaken. This is the first lesson to be learned in the pathology of acutely toxic goiters if the surgeon and his patient are to live happily ever after.

The most important phase of the surgical pathology can be learned at the operating table and there only. It has to do with the friability, not

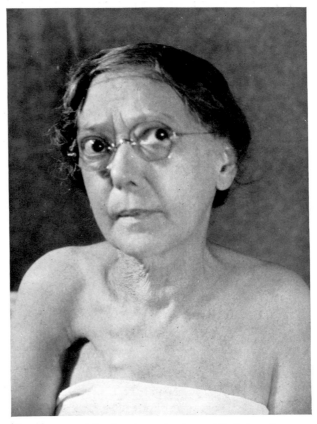

FIG. 143. Eye signs remaining in a burned-out exophthalmic goiter.

only of the thyroid capsule, but also of the vessels. The toxic gland produces a reaction in the environing connective tissue that is histochemically identical with that produced by inflammation. The result is an extreme friability of the connective tissue. The condition of the capsule when exposed at the operating table is characterized by a thickened almost edematous capsule (Fig. 144).

The very toxic gland is attached to the surrounding tissue so closely that it feels as though it were cemented. This state of affairs is com-

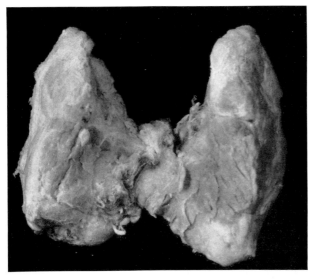

FIG. 144. Surface of a recently removed toxic goiter. The connective tissue is pale as though edematous. The fibrinous appearance of the capsule was not apparent until after dehydration.

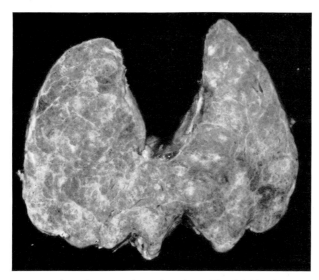

FIG. 145. Cross-section of an acutely toxic goiter. The field is divided into areas by fibrous tissue septa. The white areas mark cellular hyperplasia usually marked by extensive lymphoid infiltration.

parable with the adhesions of a chemical peritonitis. If the surgeon struggles with the difficulties associated with these changes he will appreciate the meaning of the statement, "The patient may be ready but the goiter isn't"; and he will await the subsidence of the reaction round the capsule before attempting operation.

In operating on the adherent gland one finds the thin dilated vessels are so closely attached to the surgical capsule that attempts to separate

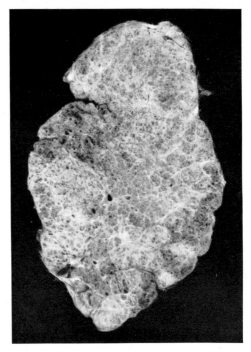

FIG. 146. Acute toxic goiter showing large vesicular acini.

them produce embarrassing hemorrhages much to the distress of the operator. Conversely, if the reaction is allowed to subside before operation, the connective tissue loses its friability and the gland can be removed from its capsule without difficulty. These facts are doubly to be emphasized since the use of Lugol's solution brings the patient in a short time to a state when she is ready, but the change in the gland is not produced so quickly. The patient may be ready for the operation but if the gland is fixed the operation should be deferred until it is removable in the surgical capsule for "The patient is ready but the gland is not." This is the most important phase in the surgical pathology of goiter. It is

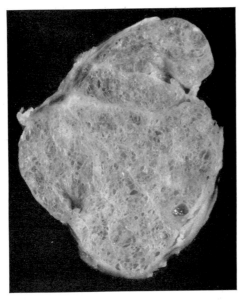

FIG. 147. Acute toxic goiter; the acini are being obliterated by cell hyperplasia.

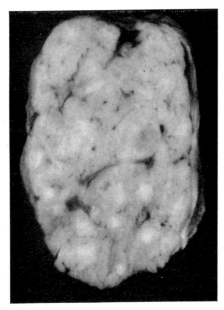

FIG. 148. Acute toxic goiter. The cut surface shows a grayish-white nearly uniform surface.

amazing to note how cheerfully the beginner will proceed with operations in cases from which the experienced operator would shrink. The mortality attests the importance of caution.

The time of permissible operation is marked by the fact that the gland becomes more mobile and is softer and less sensitive to the touch. In very toxic cases the surface of the gland feels as if it were covered with very low, firm nodulations. One cannot await the disappearance of these before undertaking operation.

The cross-section, in acute cases with slight enlargement, shows a

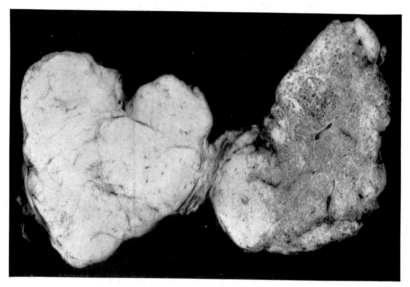

Fig. 149. Acutely toxic goiter. The right lobe is completely involved presenting a solid white surface while its fellow presents only limited areas involved.

surface divided into fields like the septa of the normal gland. Areas of cellular hyperplasia are usually marked by white firm nodules (Fig. 145). Cases in which the cellular proliferation is limited to small fields may present the gross picture of a nontoxic colloid (Fig. 146). This is particularly notable in goiters of early life when they have been preceded by a colloid stage. In older or more pronounced cases the acini are obscured by infiltration, giving the entire cut surface a whitish look (Fig. 147). In yet more acute cases marked by extremely pronounced hyperplasia the gland is very dense and the surface is white, giving the general appearance of a Hashimoto's struma (Fig. 148). In some cases one lobe only is markedly affected while the other contains wide areas which are uninvolved (Fig. 149). Such cases naturally present a greatly varying microscopic picture.

In the older patients there may be nodular formations which indicate that a simple colloid preceded the toxic state (Fig. 150). These goiters are often grayish white and are expressive of the greatest friability. Sometimes definite nodulations may be felt in the clinic which are more conspicuous on section. Some specimens show considerable structural

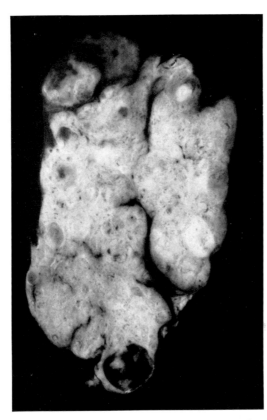

Fig. 150. Very toxic somewhat nodular goiter. F., age 48. No goiter had been noticed before the advent of exophthalmos.

variation. The mottling of the surface may be pronounced, the pale pink being interspersed with whitish nodules representing more intensive degrees of acinal proliferation (Fig. 151).

From the foregoing, therefore, it is patent that in estimating the degree of toxicity from the gross specimen one must take into account the age of the patient and the duration as well as the intensity of the symptoms. The typical acute toxic goiter in young patients may resemble the nontoxic state except for the much increased firmness to the touch. The acini may be evident to gross inspection, suggesting a limited cellular hyperplasia. Yet these goiters may be intensely toxic because it is not the number of the newly formed cells but the character of their product that determines their toxicity. One may assume that the reaction is so intense because the young are more susceptible to stimuli. In older patients, long subjects of colloid goiter, the acinal proliferation

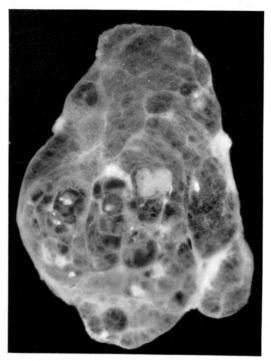

FIG. 151. Acutely toxic goiter. Definite lobulations are visible indicating a long-existing though unnoted goiter.

may be more extensive and yet the symptoms less pronounced. The difference is to be sought for in the colloid.

Histology. Despite some eminent opinions to the contrary, the histology of the acute toxic goiter is perfectly typical. Two great groups must be distinguished. Those cases which have eye signs, the exophthalmic goiters, are characterized by the formation of papillary hyperplasias which extend into the lumina of the acini. Those without eye signs are made up of acini lacking such papillations. The characteristic feature of the former is the formation of papillations extending into the

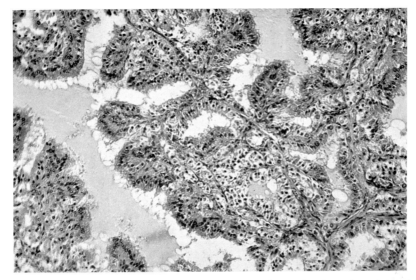

FIG. 152. Exophthalmic goiter. Papillary hyperplasias project into the acini. The colloid is crenated, retracted, palely staining. The protoplasm of some of the cells is poorly staining, others are granular indicative of great toxicity. The extensive papillations indicate a high degree of toxicity.

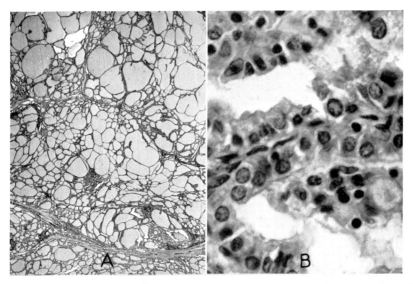

FIG. 153. Acute toxic goiter implanted on a colloid: *A*, the larger area is made up of large acini in which project new cell formations; *B*, acini lined with cuboidal epithelium. The protoplasm is sharply defined, the nuclei deeply staining, both factors indicating an active state.

lumina of the acini (Fig. 152). The papillary bearing area may form but a small part of the total goiter mass (*A*, Fig. 153), but these areas, when viewed by high power, become quite impressive (*B*, Fig. 153). In such specimens it is easy to secure pictures showing only simple acini lined with flat epithelium. Though such pictures may be from exophthalmic glands they are obviously not from the affected area. Usually the affected areas involve microscopic areas.

In some the gross appearance of the gland is that of a colloid goiter, and microscopically the large acini are lined with flat epithelium, with here and there small areas of hyperplastic acini (*A*, Fig. 154). A careless

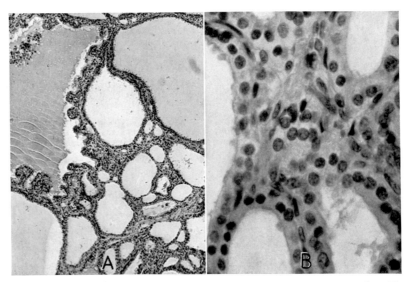

Fig. 154. Acute toxic goiter established on a simple colloid: *A*, small areas of papillary formation and newly developed acini; *B*, the cells lining the acini are low columnar, the protoplasm not sharply defined and the nuclei variously staining. The colloid is uniformly staining but pale.

microscopic study, let it be repeated, may show only such areas but if adequate study is made areas will be found showing cellular hyperplasia (*B*, Fig. 154). Sometimes an entire block removed for examination may be made up of simple acini and unless other areas are examined the real structure may be missed entirely.

The nonexophthalmic type, or stage, is characterized by the formation of simple acini without papillary formation (Fig. 155). The acini may be so small that there are few or no lumina, hence little or no colloid. Solid columns may be found. In the very toxic cases infiltration with lymph cells may be added (Fig. 156).

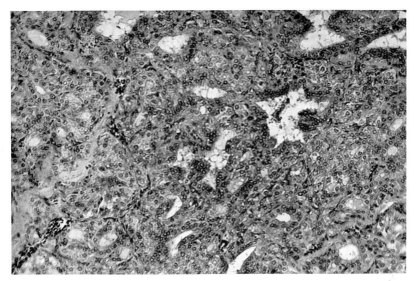

FIG. 155. Acute toxic goiter without eye signs. The entire field is made up of newly formed acini. The sparse colloid is granular or palely staining and retracted. The solid cell masses are made up of small nuclei and indefinitely outline protoplasm indicating that the proliferating capacity is dominant.

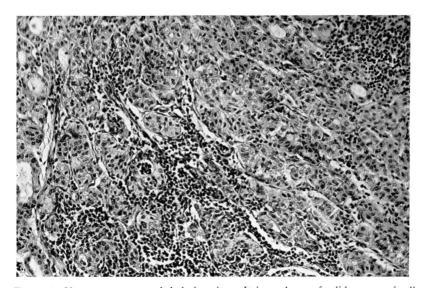

FIG. 156. Very acute nonexophthalmic goiter. It is made up of solid masses of cells almost devoid of colloid. The nuclei are small, deeply staining, the protoplasm in some areas syncytial-like. Various areas are infiltrated with lymphocytes.

In some cases a large part of the gland is formed of old acini with low epithelium interspersed with abundant interacinal connective tissue indicating an old gland (*A*, Fig. 157). Adjacent to these may be acini showing active epithelium (*B*, Fig. 157). In some of these cases the acute onset gives it the appearance of a recent process. Only the discovery of old areas makes it evident that in reality an old goiter existed before the onset of the acute symptoms. In cases in which a hypo state is encroaching on the hyper stage areas completely degenerated (*B*, Fig. 158) may dominate the field though here and there will be active areas (*A*, Fig. 158).

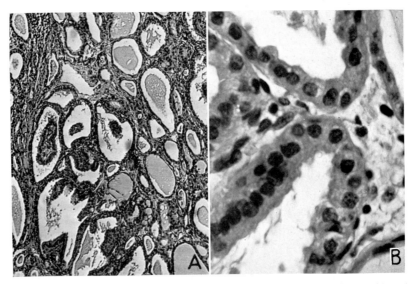

FIG. 157. Acute toxic goiter implanted on an unrecognized old colloid. *A*, Old acini lined with atrophic cells and degenerated colloid. *B*, Newly formed acini lined with columnar cells. The cells are well outlined, the nuclei uniform and deeply staining.

In both of these types unexpected failure of the heart may follow operation, marked by the sudden development of arrhythmia and in rare cases death ensues.

In very toxic cases the cells may undergo degeneration and exfoliation. This is seen particularly in cases which die unoperated on in hyperpyrexia within a short time after the beginning of the disease (Fig. 159). Mental aberration, even wild delirium, attends the final stage of this type. In most glands only certain areas are thus involved though sometimes the entire slide appears as though the tissue had been immersed in potassium hydroxide.

The colloid in acute toxic goiters is quite variable. It is generally stated that the colloid is thin. This seems likely because of the faint way in which it takes up the eosin stain. But this is by no means all. There is a granular degeneration in some areas, with the surrounding colloid taking stain faintly or not at all. If stainless with eosin the acini are called empty, obviously without reason, because it may stain with some other dye. Greater variations are demonstrable with special dyes. Mallory's methylene blue, for instance, may stain some acini orange or pale blue whereas others stain the normal deep blue. Of course the meaning of

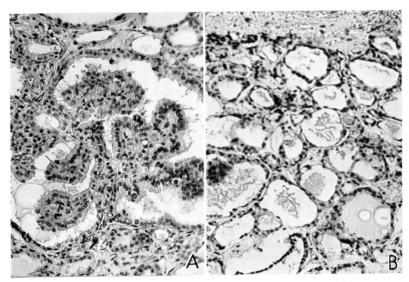

FIG. 158. Acute toxic goiter with areas of degeneration. *A*, Hyperplasia of epithelium. The colloid is sparse and granular. *B*, Acini with atrophic epithelium in part degenerated and exfoliated. The colloid is sparse and granular, in many acini reduced to the point of disappearance.

these tinctorial variations is not known, but since certain tinctorial changes harmonize with variations in clinical phenomena their study may ultimately lead to a more complete understanding of the change involved.

What comes of that part of the gland one leaves at operation? Some writers believe the acinal epithelium returns to normal. They come to this conclusion after examination of material obtained at autopsy in patients previously operated on and definitely cured. My own material has been limited to tissue removed at recurrences and that obtained after removing the second lobe some months subsequent to the removal of the first in a two stage operation. Also in those cases in which recovery is not satisfactory after a conservative operation and one proceeds to another operation removing the remaining part of the gland. The structure is similar to that of the material obtained at the first operation. Such operations show also that a small nodule of gland may keep up the toxic symptoms and that unsatisfactory results from operation are due to the fact that a part of the disease was allowed to remain, because of the fear of post-operative myxedema.

I have studied particularly those cases in which the operation was done in two stages. One lobe removed, the patient improves markedly. The second lobe removed—in two months or two years, it matters little —after unquestioned pronounced clinical improvement, the tissues show

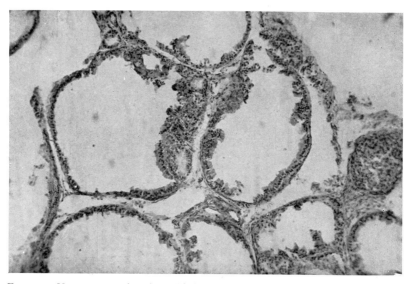

FIG. 159. Very acute toxic goiter. Died unoperated on in wild delirium, temperature 107°. The epithelium is degenerated, in part exfoliated, even the septa are destroyed. The colloid is pale, abundant but indifferent.

the same cellular structure. What change there is must be sought in the colloid (Fig. 160). It stains more deeply, is more uniform and fills out the acini more completely. Some cellular changes in the cells are occasionally found; the cell protoplasm in the first lobe removed may stain less intensely than that in the second, but there is no move on the part of the epithelium to return to normal. It continues columnar and the papillations remain. Of course if only a single block is studied great variation may be found but if the study be thorough there seems to be little difference. This is rather confusing because great improvement may follow the first operation and one would think this would be reflected in the structure of the epithelium of the remaining gland.

Generally speaking, the histologic changes are in proportion to the clinical manifestations of the disease but this is by no means universally so. Pronounced clinical signs may be associated with relatively slight changes. The type of cell change is more nearly directly associated with the clinical signs than the extent. That is to say, in some cases only small areas may be involved in the Basedow papillation but these small areas can show an intense cell activity. The greater part of the gland may show a simple colloid goiter. The younger the patient the more likely is this to be the case. If in the clinic apparently very toxic cases show

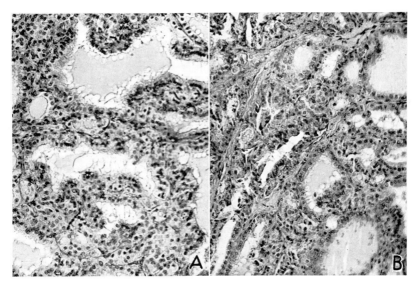

FIG. 160. Acute toxic goiter. *A*, Slide from first lobe removed. Cells palely staining, the protoplasm pale, degenerated. *B*, Second lobe removed three months later. The cells stain well and the colloid is more uniform and deeply staining, except in some of the smaller acini.

less cell proliferation than one expects much light may be thrown on the problem by studying anew the clinical manifestations and the course immediately after operation. A consideration of these may show that the patient was not really so toxic as one at first thought. The follow-up of the patient may show that there was a basic nervous state which led us astray. One must not look to the slide for confirmation of clinical errors.

Literature

Toxic Diffuse Goiters. The literature of acute toxic goiter is so confused that the young surgeon is more apt to be bewildered than instructed by much reading. The best reading is to be found in the slide. I would advise the young surgeon to observe three patients of the diffuse toxic without eye signs and three typical exophthalmic goiters in the clinic and then secure slides from each of the goiters and study each of these carefully, say three hours a day for a month or two. Then he can read the following and he will be relatively immune from the confusion of the literature: Wilson (*Northwestern Med.*, Jan. 1913, 1–5; *Med. Rec.*, Aug. 1913, 84, 373–378; *Am. J. Med. Sc.*, Dec. 1913, 156, 781; *J. Michigan State Med. Soc.*, Sept. 1922, 21, 369–373); Lewis (*Am. J. Med. Sc.* Jan. 1931, 181, 65) and Hellwig (*Surg., Gynec. and Obst.*, Aug. 1928, 47, 173; *ibid.*, Jan. 1931, 52, 43–51.)

CHAPTER X

Thyroiditis

INFLAMMATIONS of the thyroid gland are fairly common and present a wide range of lesions. In the first place the previously normal gland may be affected or there may be a pre-existing goiter. In the second place there are frank infections easily aligned with similar lesions in other tissues. These latter are definitely microbic and are to be distinguished from the lesions established on pre-existing goiters in which it has been impossible to establish a microbic origin. It is well for our understanding not to emphasize too much the inflammatory nature of the last named group because its clinical importance lies in a wholly different direction.

Inflammations of a previously goitrous gland are very rare. True inflammations which usually involve a previously nongoitrous gland are generally divided into the nonsuppurative and the suppurative. This division is justified by their life history. However, they have much in common, so much in truth that many authors do not distinguish between them and as a matter of fact a distinction cannot be made in some cases until the disease has run its course. Therefore it is sometimes convenient to regard them as synonymous when one does not know whether or not there will be suppuration in a particular case. However, when one contemplates the terrible viciousness of the suppurative form one cannot help but place it in a separate category; certainly we do so in retrospect.

The lesions not so frankly inflammatory can be established on a previously goitrous gland but may possibly involve a previously normal gland. The former plays its rôle within the gland and is characterized by extensive infiltration by lymph cells, first accurately described by Hashimoto and commonly designated by his name. The other, first adequately described by Riedel, extends beyond the gland and is commonly designated by his name. The latter is regarded by some authors as the final stage of the former. To confuse the two seems to me preposterous when viewed from the clinical point of view, and I believe it is possible to distinguish between them from the slide alone. Judging from the ultimate results, I believe Riedel's struma is more closely related to nonsuppurative thyroiditis than to Hashimoto's struma.

The first, Hashimoto's disease, confines itself to the gland and leaves the capsule uninvolved. This, the much more common form, in my experience, remains such throughout.   Its chief interest lies in its close relationship to myxedema.

Riedel's struma, on the contrary, invades the capsule and wide areas beyond in a manner that is amazing, even incredible in extreme cases. In my experience I have found it already extended beyond the gland when the patient first came under observation.   So constantly is this true that one can say in the clinic that if it does not already extend beyond the capsule it will not do so.   I have encountered no exceptions.

These various clinical pictures may be studied under the following heads:

    I.   Acute Nonsuppurative Thyroiditis
   II.   Acute Suppurative Thyroiditis
  III.   Chronic Lymphatic Thyroiditis (Hashimoto's Thyroiditis)
  IV.   Chronic Nonspecific Thyroiditis (Riedel's Struma)

One can make a group of the chronic specific thyroiditides, or granulomas, to include tuberculosis and syphilis but since I have seen only two cases of tuberculosis, and did not recognize either one until the slide was examined, and have seen none at all of syphilis, a discussion of these diseases is omitted.

ACUTE NONSUPPURATIVE THYROIDITIS

In this type there are evidences of acute inflammation and it may develop in thyroids which have not been the previous site of a goiter. This type is not infrequently an accompaniment of a great variety of acute infectious diseases.   The frequency of this association, notably with typhoid fever, makes it seem likely that it is bacterial in nature, obviously not of the pus producing type and probably not due to any particular organism.   Be this as it may, this conception helps one to understand the clinical course.

The disease is characterized by a relatively mild course and subsides spontaneously within several weeks.   Because of the mild onset one can recognize it as belonging to the nonsuppurative type.   It can be compared to postoperative parotiditis, causing much focal disturbance but seldom ending in suppuration.   In some cases the inflammation lingers and ultimately an abscess forms.   Commonly enough it is observed as an isolated lesion unaccompanied by any other disease.

Pathogenesis.   The initiatory symptoms are those of local inflammation.   A painful area in the front of the neck is usually the first symptom. General constitutional symptoms are seldom notable and are often entirely absent.   There is moderate swelling which is painful to the touch and hot to the feel. Usually there is a moderate rise of temperature accompanied by the general symptoms of loss of appetite, general malaise, with some loss of weight in the severer cases.

The height of the process usually lasts only a few weeks; then the temperature begins to subside and the tenderness to abate. Complete resolution, however, usually requires many weeks. If the course is prolonged it is well to keep them in mind, for sometimes an abscess forms late in the disease, particularly in the aged and feeble. In such cases the

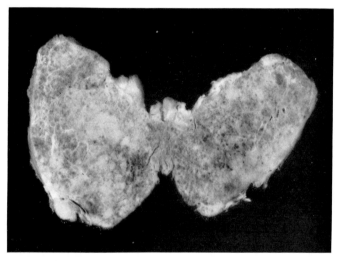

Fig. 161. Late stage of acute nonsuppurative thyroiditis. Acini distinguishable in most areas but in some replaced by fibrous tissue.

abscess may find an exit through the skin, into the esophagus, or it may burrow into the tissues of the neck without an acute exacerbation being evident. These cases belong, of course, to the rarities.

Old colloid goiters seldom develop an abscess. Usually these follow hemorrhage into a nodule which gradually involves the skin and is followed by an indolent abscess. These belong to the degenerative processes rather than to the inflammations.

Material for study is all too scarce, but it seems that the final stage is a more or less pronounced fibrosis with associated involvement of the parenchymal tissue. Such tissues are seldom available for study because one must see these cases in the clinic, but sometimes the history of the past disease is highly suggestive, and then the gland must be secured after the disease subsides.

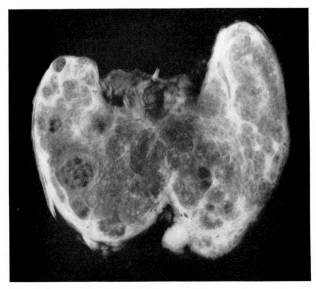

Fig. 162. End stage of nonsuppurative thyroiditis. The thyroid tissue is surrounded and displaced by newly formed connective tissue.

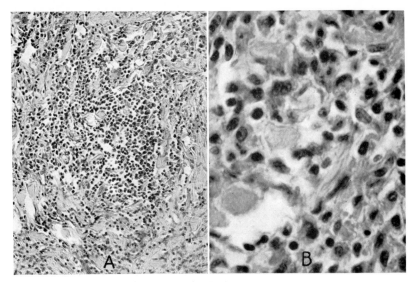

Fig. 163. Acute nonsuppurative thyroiditis, late stage: *A*, fibrosis intermingled with numerous round cells; *B*, high power; newly formed fibers, fibroblasts with large ovoid palely staining nuclei and round cells deeply staining. The acini are degenerated, marked by only a few poorly staining cells.

Pathology. The hardness and fixity associated with marked tenderness bespeak an inflammatory induration. The inflammation is confined within the capsule but the latter participates sufficiently to fix the gland to the surrounding structures. The edema about the inflamed gland usually is not so extensive but that the outline of the organ can be distinctly made out. The feel is occasionally simulated by some acutely toxic goiters, the difference being that in the inflammatory lesions there is no evidence of hypersecretion, though of course an acutely inflamed

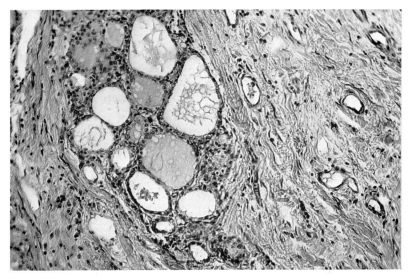

FIG. 164. Terminal stage of acute nonsuppurative thyroiditis. Dense fibrous tissue with few intensely staining nuclei. Numerous prominent blood vessels. A group of acini with well preserved cuboidal epithelium. Colloid thin and degenerated.

thyroid gland is not conducive to tranquillity and a toxic goiter is sometimes diagnosed when none really exists.

Usually these glands are not operated on since they resolve in the course of weeks. If operation is attempted the capsule is found to be very little edematous and attachment to the surrounding muscles is not marked.

The cross-section generally presents an intense red surface but later in the course of the disease there may be mottled white areas (Fig. 161). It is likely that such cases are really examples of Hashimoto's disease. Other cases show a true fibrosis distributed throughout the gland and dividing it into fields. The fibrous areas are dense, heavy bundles. In some cases, surrounding degenerated areas of the gland, pronounced formation of fibrous tissue develops (Fig. 162). This may invade the surrounding muscle layers and be quite indistinguishable from Riedel's struma except that it is localized near the area of degeneration.

Histology. The microscopic structure is that of a normal or goitrous gland area, between the acini of which there is intense round cell and polynuclear infiltration (Fig. 163). The connective tissue may be swollen and stain faintly with acid dyes. The colloid is palely staining, and the polynuclear infiltration provides the distinguishing sign. The end stage is characterized by heavy fibrous bands and in some areas an atrophic acinal epithelium (Fig. 164). These glands resemble the atrophied ones occasionally seen in myxedemics.

ACUTE SUPPURATING THYROIDITIS

As noted above, suppuration sometimes occurs late in the group generally classed as nonsuppurative. The really acute suppurative type is something quite different. In these the onset is commonly so stormy that the constitutional symptoms overshadow the local lesion and the latter is overlooked until a burrowing abscess has formed. So often is this true that I have come to investigate the thyroid region in cases when a hyperacute infectious process is at hand, the nature of which is not apparent. I determined on this precaution because I have seen more of these cases in the autopsy room, previously unrecognized, than in the clinic. In some cases, however, when the infection is mild and particularly in those which develop during the course of some infectious disease, such as pneumonia or typhoid fever, the onset may be less acute and proceed more leisurely to the formation of an abscess. It is these that present the border-line between the nonsuppurative and the suppurative, and that are, as noted above, likely produced by other than the usual pyogenic organisms. With the type now under consideration we have to do with pus producing organisms, sometimes even with mixed infections.

This acute suppurative variety often begins with high fever and chills; sometimes, especially in children, with delirium. So violent may be the onset, let it be repeated, that there is no localization of the complaint. In those beginning less violently there is pain which is often referred to the mastoid region or the occiput rather than the thyroid region, and when accompanied by contraction of the neck muscles and delirium it may lead the clinician astray. Occasionally the picture is that of an acute abdominal crisis with retraction and rigidity of the abdominal muscles. I once saw a surgeon of national reputation do a laparotomy for a supposedly acute abdominal crisis. The thyroid abscess was first discovered at autopsy. I saw such glaring errors in my pathology days that I had not the courage to acquaint the clinician with my findings at the autopsy. I have a suspicion that a similar feeling has kept much interesting material out of the literature; at any rate I have not seen the attending surgeon rush into print in such cases.

In rare instances the onset is so impetuous that the delirium may be very severe and prolonged with the result that the thyroid inflammation is overlooked and a brain lesion is suspected. The mental agitation in one case I saw was so great that the patient was sent to an asylum under a diagnosis of acute mania. The thyroid infection was not discovered until the abscess pointed in the suprasternal notch two months later. In days gone by it was not uncommon for the thyroid trouble to go unnoticed, a typhoid fever being diagnosed. Some of the cases reported in the literature as thyroid suppuration following typhoid fever may have been thyroiditis and nothing else.

Not all cases are so severe. Pain and swelling in the thyroid region may be immediately obvious, resembling in this the nonsuppurating type, and the differential diagnosis may be in doubt for a time. Usually the surrounding tissues are so much infiltrated that the outline of the gland cannot be distinctly made out. This evidence usually permits a differentiation from the nonsuppurative type early in the course of the disease. Later on the skin becomes intensely reddened and the tenderness becomes more localized. This is evidence enough that an abscess lies beneath and it is a signal that drainage is required. Burrowing into undesirable places usually precedes fluctuation and proclaims lack of clinical acumen.

With the local signs constitutional reactions are in evidence. The leukocytosis is in harmony with the nature of the process. Commonly the temperature is high. The typical temperature curve, once the disease is established, is distinctly septic. The most exquisite picket fence curve I have ever seen was in a case of acute suppurating thyroiditis. It continued between subnormal and 104° for more than five weeks, with the most astonishing regularity, before a threatening perforation of a neck abscess called attention to the true state of affairs.

Neglected, the abscess seeks its own outlet, sometimes on the surface; but more common than a skin fistula is perforation into the esophagus, or, less often, into the trachea; in the latter case the results may be immediately disastrous. I once had a patient embarrass me by developing a fistula simultaneously into the esophagus and through the skin so that the fluids he swallowed escaped through the external orifice. In very old patients not carefully watched the formation of such an abscess may easily be overlooked.

Obviously, therefore, if the induration of the gland is great a considerable abscess must be formed before fluctuation is discovered. In fact fluctuation should not be awaited in any case. When there are pronounced symptoms as above enumerated in the presence of a hard thyroid, exploration will discover an abscess. Once the abscess is drained recovery is rapid and complete unless neglect has permitted the infection to extend into the mediastinum.

Pathology. The hard indurated gland with pronounced subcutaneous edema is about all that is ascertainable in the early cases. Thyroidectomies naturally are not done in this condition. The material obtained by incision brings forth a granular friable tissue.

Unfortunately autopsies furnish material enough for the study of terminal pathology. The abscesses may occupy one or both lobes. They may be multiple, and astonishingly small in view of the symptoms they produce. On the other hand, the entire gland may be destroyed. Some writers have designated this as gangrene, but the term is justified only when the entire lobe dies simultaneously, not when the destruction results from the confluence of many abscesses advancing from center to periphery. If there is any thyroid tissue surrounding the abscess it is intensely red and firm unless softened by the abscess.

The bacteria contained in these abscesses present a varying flora, the staphylococcus being the most common in the serious cases. The crude technic of a surgical pathologist may fail to demonstrate any bacteria in the long existing cases. Usually, however, he finds too many.

Histology. The slide of such a tissue presents a connective tissue intensely infiltrated with polynuclear cells. Remains of acini with exfoliated epithelium may be found at some distance from the abscess wall.

CHRONIC LYMPHATIC THYROIDITIS (HASHIMOTO'S THYROIDITIS, STRUMA LYMPHOMATOSA, LYMPHADENITIS-JOLL)

Like most diseases we do not understand, that now under discussion is burdened with many names. The designation here adopted, suggested by Gordon Lee, is in a measure descriptive and is free from the dissonance of struma lymphomatosa which has a foreign sound. In the study of many glands one finds small lymphoid areas scattered here and there. These differ from the lymph follicles commonly found in certain types of glands but are characterized by invasion of the interacinal connective tissue. The consequence is a change in the epithelium which results in obliteration of the acini. The term applied by Joll, lymphadenitis, seems to point in the right direction, but since the disease is a progressive one the term used to head this chapter seems preferable because it is more comprehensive.

Why the disease goes on to such fibrosing chronicity is unknown. It is something more than a nonspecific thyroiditis fortuitously characterized by the presence of lymphoid tissue, because lymph cells dominate and often there are distinct follicles, germinal areas and all, but we must reflect that these may have been present before the disease began. Because of its very definite clinical picture it is sometimes confused with the nonsuppurative thyroiditis on one hand and with Riedel's struma on the other. The outcome in both, it must be remembered, is the same: the formation of keloid-like tissue. The associated cellular change, which has acquired a new interest since its relation to myxedema seems to be close, is not found in Riedel's struma.

It is generally assumed that this disease is always established on a pre-existing goiter. However, in many cases the patients are not aware that they had goiters before the onset of the disease; and the anatomic study of the gland sometimes reveals no evidence of a pre-existent enlargement.

The disease is relatively slow in onset. The gland becomes gradually larger; it is tender and firm but still retains the outline of the normal organ. It scarcely involves the gland capsule and never extends beyond it. It is characterized by infiltration of the thyroid gland by many lymphocytes; on this point all are agreed. Equally obvious, it seems to me, are the changes in the acinal epithelium. In fact the changes in the epithelium are so unfailing that one suspects that this may be the initiatory lesion. Some writers believe the disease is a local manifestation of a constitutional disease. This cannot be because a complete thyroidectomy entirely eliminates it.

If one keeps the essential features of the disease in mind small localized lesions will often be recognized which, because of their limited extent, are not usually recognized as Hashimoto's struma.

The surgeon's chief interest in this disease lies in the fact that it is very commonly the forerunner of myxedema and the peculiar changes in the acinal epithelium may apprise the surgeon of the fact that the patient will manifest a postoperative hypo state before manifesting the symptoms.

This association between Hashimoto's disease and myxedema has been so generally recognized that surgeons have advised either no operation at all or the removal of only just sufficient tissue to relieve respiratory disturbance. Yet the truth is that the presence of this type of goiter indicates complete removal is imperative in order to avert the hypo state. This fact warrants the hypothesis that the hypo state is due to the action of the acinal cells characteristic of this disease.

Pathogenesis. The significant thing about this type of thyroiditis is that it is most prevalent in women at about the menopause, which suggests an endocrine relationship though there is no evidence of a direct association with disturbance of any other endocrine organ.

The patient seeks the surgeon because a goiter has appeared or because an already existing goiter has rapidly enlarged and become more sensitive to pressure. There may be few or no general disturbances. Later deglutition may be interfered with and breathing be impaired.

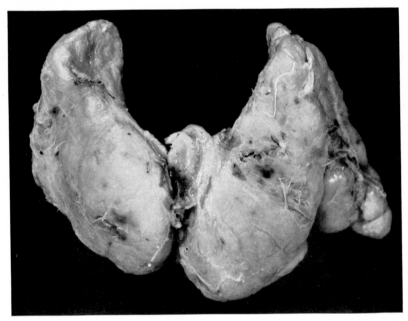

FIG. 165. Chronic lymphatic thyroiditis (Hashimoto's). Removed by total thyroidectomy. The goiter was white, smooth and very hard.

The constitutional signs are not pronounced; the nervousness and loss of weight, if any, are due to the local disturbance. There is no evidence of hyperthyroidism.

The disease is notable for the absence of symptoms of increased toxicity, nervousness and loss of weight except as above noted. This is important because the physical characteristics closely resemble those of a very toxic gland though there is no evidence of hyperthyroidism.

The disease is slow in onset and of prolonged course. In fact the course continues to the final stage which is fibrosis and degeneration of acinal epithelium.

The fact is that these cases, at least most of them, terminate in spontaneous myxedema. Curiously enough this fact, above noted, has persuaded many surgeons to eschew removal of the usual amount of tissue. My own reaction is that since the condition ends in myxedema this consequence may be obviated by removing the entire gland. Clinical experience appears to confirm this opinion.

The important fact, it seems to me, is that the changes characteristic of Hashimoto's disease are found in many old goiters which never experienced the characteristic changes of the typical case. If an old goiter

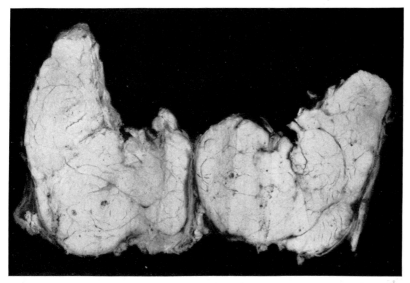

Fig. 166. Cross-section of a chronic lymphatic thyroiditis (Hashimoto's). The surface is diffusely grayish white.

has become hard, though only in some areas, such changes must be suspected and met by a very radical operation.

Pathology. The physical findings are those of a hard gland, like acute toxic goiter, but there is no evidence of hyperthyroidism. The increase in sensitiveness may be such as to excite comment. The goiter is very hard, suggesting malignancy, but the gland is uniformly enlarged and withal movable and the onset usually is more rapid than in malignant tumors.

When the operation is undertaken the capsule is found slightly if at all adherent; the hemorrhage is not likely to be notable, but because of the uniform hardness of the gland anything less than a total 'ectomy may be difficult. The surface is generally smooth but sometimes moderately bosselated (Fig. 165). The color is whitish gray. The firmness of the gland at operation is even more impressive than in the clinic.

The cross-section is quite white or grayish white or mottled white and red, giving an almost translucent appearance in some areas (Fig. 166). The surface shows division into lobules by bands of white or pinkish white connective tissue but in the fibrosing end stage this differentiation is lost.

It is necessary to include numerous atypical cases in the group of chronic lymphatic thyroiditis. In many nodular goiters areas are found

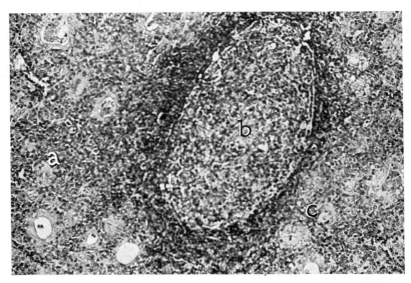

FIG. 167. Lymph nodule with germinal center in early chronic lymphatic thyroiditis: *a*, follicles surrounded by lymphatic infiltration; *b*, lymph follicle with germinal center; *c*, acini obliterated by the infiltration, the cells of which are palely staining.

which may be regarded as local forms of the disease. In such cases a localized white nodule may be in evidence but sometimes the local manifestations are less obvious, being expressed more by a hardness than a change in color. This type is important because while clinical evidence of the disease may be lacking the slide shows the typical changes. A postoperative myxedema may be expected in such cases. In fact if the clinical course be carefully studied it will be discovered that most postoperative hypo states were in evidence before the operation was performed.

Histology. The essential feature of this disease that is usually emphasized is the intense infiltration of the interacinal spaces with lymphocytes. These may be diffusely distributed in the interacinal tissue or may

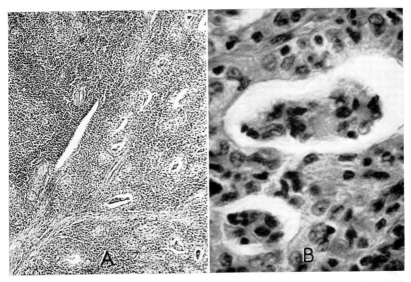

FIG. 168. Chronic lymphatic thyroiditis: *A*, intense lymphatic infiltration all but obliterating the acini; *B*, acini in which the epithelium is exfoliated into a cavity devoid of demonstrable colloid. The exfoliated epithelium is in a state of degeneration.

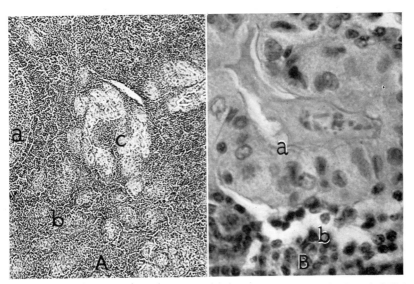

FIG. 169. Chronic lymphatic thyroiditis: *A*, low power, *a*, edge of a lymph follicle; *b*, intense lymph cell infiltration; *c*, acini filled with large foamy cells; *B*, high power, *a*, large illy staining cells sometimes mistaken for metastases of adrenal tumors; *b*, lymph cells.

form lymph follicles, germinal centers and all (Fig. 167). The cellular infiltration may be so great that the acini are entirely hidden (*A*, Fig. 168) but usually they appear as small lumina in an otherwise cellular area. In such intense cases the acinal epithelium may be exfoliated (*B*, Fig. 168).

The fundamental feature of the disease, it seems to me, is to be found in the acinal cells. They are large and foamy (Fig. 169) and fill the entire acinal cavity. The acini are free of colloid. Quite striking are the cases in which the acinal cells form clumps without any lumina at all. This is a constant feature of the disease and is sufficient alone to distinguish it from the other forms discussed in this chapter. Furthermore, when one sees these cells in the slide one may be sure that the patient will have a postoperative myxedema. The connective tissue may be swollen, stain faintly, have few nuclei. The connective tissue changes differ from that of Riedel's struma which is marked by the formation of heavy keloid-like bundles which are always absent in the Hashimoto type, at least until the terminal stages.

CHRONIC NONSPECIFIC THYROIDITIS (RIEDEL'S STRUMA)

The intracapsular thyroiditis described in the preceding section is sometimes confused with Riedel's struma, but only by those who have never seen a real Riedel's struma at the operating table. The former plays its rôle within the thyroid capsule and the goiter is always movable. Riedel's struma, on the contrary, involves the capsule and in extreme cases extends far beyond the confines of the goiter, involving the adjacent muscles of the neck, the connective tissue and even the carotid sheath. A good clinical synonym is "woody phlegmon involving the thyroid gland."

Pathogenesis. The onset, in the cases I have observed, has not been acute. The patient relates that there has been a gradual swelling about the neck, not particularly painful but causing a sense of constriction, of suffocation, sometimes limiting the flexion of the head. The entire front of the neck, in fact, comes to be occupied by a diffuse swelling, firm, hard, woody, actually equal to the woody phlegmon of the neck not associated with the thyroid gland. The swelling may extend far beyond the sterno-mastoid muscles, to the occiput and even into the medastinum.

The severe cases involve the entire gland and form a hard collar about the neck. Minor cases may involve only one lobe or even only a part of a lobe. In fact in routine examinations of thyroid glands one occasionally finds an area of keloid connective tissue which seems to be the final stage of a Riedel's struma which was unsuspected in the absence of a history suggesting any considerable disturbance. In clinically recognizable cases one may find areas of thyroid tissue, goitrous or otherwise, within the confines of the Riedel's struma. So confined the disturbance may not be important except for the increased difficulty experienced at the operating table. This is in contrast with the more extensive cases in which radical operation is impossible.

In the bilateral cases the sense of suffocation increases; dyspnea, even cyanosis may develop necessitating an emergency exposure of the trachea.

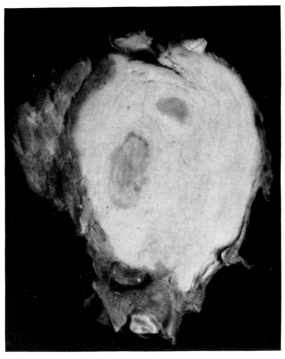

FIG. 170. Chronic nonspecific thyroiditis (Riedel's struma). The mass is white, very hard, enclosing in the center some but slightly affected thyroid tissue. The surface of the mass shows extraglandular tissue it was necessary to remove.

Deglutition is interfered with and may even become impossible. With all this there is little or no constitutional disturbance, the attendant loss of weight corresponding to the difficulty of taking nourishment.

Having attained its height the disease remains stationary for weeks, even many months, and then gradually subsides and in the course of from three to nine months finally disappears leaving only a sclerosed gland. It seems that myxedema does not follow Riedel's struma even though nothing but a mass of fibrous tissue remains after the disease has run its course. Unfortunately little effort appears to have been made to determine the fate of the patient or the gland after the disease has run its course.

Some surgeons attempt to remove the disease en masse in their first case. This is good news to the pathologist but the operation is usually so incomplete that the result had best be designated a biopsy. On the other hand those localized in one lobe may be removed without difficulty, albeit with the loss of some adjacent tissue. One is content in the more

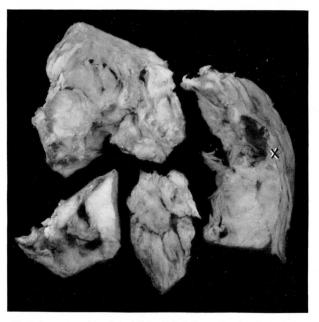

FIG. 171. Chronic nonspecific thyroiditis (Riedel's struma). Only parts of the mass could be removed. The mass at the right, *x*, has attached an overlying muscle. (R. Y. Jones' case.)

serious cases, when one must interfere, with exposure of the trachea sufficiently to relieve the urgent symptoms and with removing what biopsy material his pathologic curiosity compels. The cut surface in such cases is white and the cut vessels show as round lumina, the nature of the tissue preventing the collapse of the vessel walls.

Pathology. The hard fixed mass gives one a shock when first palpated. The density gives the impression of a huge carcinoma but the hard area ends gradually in the sides of the neck, the subcutaneous tissue being everywhere hard. The border of the tumor lacks the small hard bossela-

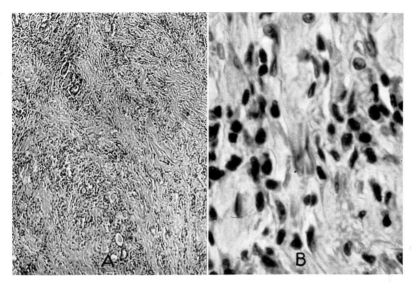

FIG. 172. Active stage of chronic nonsuppurative thyroiditis (Riedel's struma). *A*, The mass is made up of newly formed fibrous tissue with a few acini below. *B*, Fiber bundles interspersed with large deeply staining cells round and spindle-form.

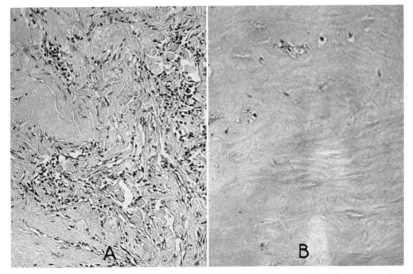

FIG. 173. Chronic nonsuppurative thyroiditis. *A*, Late but still active stage. Large keloid-like bundles with few, mostly spindleform cells with a few clusters of ovoid cells. The small vessels are surrounded by round cells. *B*, The end stage only fibrous tissue with scarcely any nuclei.

tions characteristic of cancer. However, the difference may not be apparent until a cross-section is made.

Fortunately, I have never obtained autopsy material but such has seemed at times to be imminently available. All the tissue in the extreme cases cannot be obtained at operation. In minor cases the entire gland can be removed (Fig. 170) but in the severer cases one must be content with partial removal (Fig. 171). With this material it is possible to trace the invasion, even in the gross, of the adjacent muscle and connective tissue. At the operating table it has all the characteristics of a keloid mass.

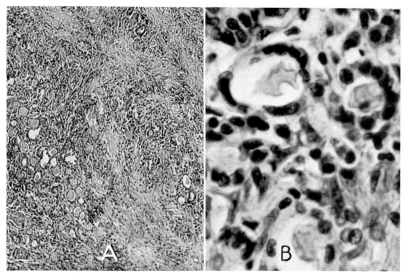

Fig. 174. Chronic nonsuppurative thyroiditis: *A*, despite extensive formation of fibrous tissue the acini are well preserved and contain some colloid; *B*, high power showing the relation of the fibrous tissue to the acini. Some acinal cells are completely degenerated.

The cut surface is white—whiter than the cut surface of a carcinoma —and is uniform, lacking the granulations evident in cancer. It is less friable, and cuts with a creaking sound quite different from the easy cutting of malignancy. The surface is bloodless, the smaller vessels being compressed by the exudate. Large vessels on the other hand may be held patulous by the induration. Bleeding from these is hard to control because of the density of the tissue. This fact, together with the extensive infiltration, is what usually changes the surgeon's mind and ends a proposed 'ectomy in a biopsy.

Histology. The slide of Riedel's disease is entirely different from one of Hashimoto's disease. Lymph cell infiltration which is characteristic

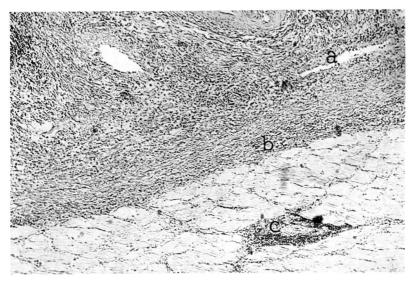

FIG. 175. Chronic nonsuppurative thyroiditis. The extraglandular tissue is being invaded; *a*, acini with capsular blood vessel; *b*, invasion of the gland capsule; *c*, muscle fibers being infiltrated by connective tissue cells, and are edematous.

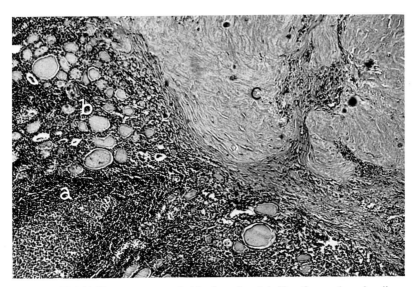

FIG. 176. Keloid-like area surrounded by lymph cell infiltration: *a*, lymph cell mass with germinal center compressing the adjacent acini; *b*, well preserved acini with colloid; *c*, keloid-like fibrous tissue almost completely devoid of cells.

of the latter is absent in the former. There is instead the formation of heavy fiber bundles which dominate the field (Fig. 172). In the earlier stages the fibrosis is active, characterized by newly formed fibrous tissue bundles and many large deeply staining ovoid cells. As the process ages these cells are less conspicuous. Later on there remain only heavy bundles of fibrous tissue which stains like keloid fibers and the cells are sparse (*A*, Fig. 173). At the end the cells have all but vanished (*B*, Fig. 173).

Even more characteristic is the difference in the acinal cells in the two diseases. In Riedel's the acinal epithelium, even when surrounded by new fibrous tissue, is preserved, when not actually compressed by the newly formed connective tissue and a fairly normal colloid fills the acini (Fig. 174). In the early stage the numerous round cells have caused confusion. When these surround a blood vessel they give the picture of a sarcoma and obviously sometimes are reported as such. Other areas may show a few leukocytes and polynuclear cells which aid in the diagnosis. Whatever the disease may be it is neither a true inflammation, nor a true tumor.

At the border of the tumor the adjacent tissues are invaded by the fibroplastic cells (Fig. 175). These cells invade the muscle tissue for a considerable distance suggesting very much the invasion of sarcoma cells.

In routine examination of goiters one sometimes comes across small sclerotic areas of keloid-like connective tissue (Fig. 176). When surrounded by areas of lymph cells it suggests Hashimoto's struma. Of course lymph follicles are found in many goiters without otherwise having any particular significance, though this may indicate some relationship between the two diseases. Since the nature of the fibers suggest Riedel's struma one is in doubt which was active. In such cases the final stages meet in the laboratory.

Literature

Thyroiditis. The preceding account is based on my own clinical experience. There is much more to be said. Crotti (Thyroid and Thymus, Lea and Febiger, ed. 2, 1922) and Joll (Diseases of the Thyroid Gland, Mosby, 1932) contain excellent accounts of everything that has happened, and then some. The latter particularly presents a clear description. This is especially true in distinguishing between Riedel's disease and lymphadenoid goiter—which I take to be synonymous with Hashimoto's disease—and which is a better term.

The nonsuppurative inflammations are described in the classic by de Quervain (Die akute, nicht eiterige Thyreoiditis, Mitt. a. d. Grenzgeb. d. Med. u. Chir., Supplement 2, 1904, 1–64). This still presents everything that is known, though it takes in some cases now better recognized as chronic lymphoid thyroiditis.

Bohan (M. Clin. N. Amer., 1924, 7, 1069–1074) suggests bad teeth as the etiologic factor in a case of thyroid inflammation. This implication is safe, for infected teeth like high taxes may be condemned in any discussion and no voice will be raised asking for proof. As a matter of fact the source of infection and the avenue of its entrance are not known. Joll (l c.) lists a large number of diseases associated with thyroiditis. Definite bacteriologic evidence is lacking except perhaps in the case of the pneumococcus and the typhoid bacillus.

CHAPTER XI

Myxedema

MYXEDEMA is a clinical term signifying a myxoid edema of the subcutaneous tissues. It is presumably due to a lack of thyroid secretion. This opinion is based on the fact that the condition is ameliorated by giving thyroid extract. This represents about the sum total of our knowledge and has in a measure closed our eyes to some very obvious facts. It should first of all be realized that the word is not synonymous with deficient thyroid secretion. It is important to keep this in mind because there can be a deficiency or an absence of thyroid secretion without any clinical signs of myxedema as total thyroidectomies have shown. Nor is myxedema the superlative degree of thyroid dysfunction or the physical expression thereof. In cases in which myxedema is associated with a hyperthyroid state we have a combined minus and a plus state. This emphasizes the paucity of our fundamental knowledge.

Myxedema is a clinical term and is expressive only of advanced states. The recognition of minor degrees of the disease is still a matter of the future. That there is a pre- or a submyxoid state, possibly a stage, there can be no doubt. In order to understand the lesser disturbances we need to mobilize all our resources. The study of the pathology together with the clinical state is requisite for even an approximately correct interpretation of many of the obscurer phases of the disease. Having exhausted our resources, constant observation of the patient may be necessary to confirm the correctness of our conclusions.

On the other hand we are prone to anticipate a deficient thyroid secretion in circumstances in which our theories lead us to expect such deficiency, notably after operations during which larger amounts of the gland are removed than we regard as safe. If any untoward signs develop following operation thyroid medication is at once resorted to. If the use of thyroid substance ameliorates the condition which he had anticipated the surgeon is prone to believe that it was caused by deficiency and by that alone. He concludes that the unfortunate state might have been prevented by a less radical operation. Thus conscience doth make cowards of us all, or at least it has done so.

This chapter is an attempt to view the whole subject from the standpoint of clinial experience, reinforced by that of the laboratory, without any reference to preconceived notions. Such re-examination is now possible since we have freed ourselves from the taboo of too radical operating and do not hesitate at complete removal of the thyroid in spontaneous myxedema.

The disease is generally divided into a spontaneous type and a secondary one that results from a too radical operation on the thyroid gland. That is the orthodox way of expressing the problem. Better stated they are divisible into cases depending on an imperfectly understood pathologic state, and those first recognized after a thyroidectomy has been performed. To admit, even insist, that myxedema following operation is due to the removal of too much of the gland is to throw the cards on the table for the attorney for the plaintiff. This is poor law and worse science. There is not a particle of warrant for such an admission.

If we limit our concept to what we know it is immediately obvious that a hypo state may have preceded the operation, and would have developed further whether the patient had been operated on or not. Furthermore there is evidence that a more radical operation might have prevented the development of a myxedema. If the surgeon is culpable it is because he removed too little rather than too much.

While myxedema is relatively common in this country, its juvenile prototype, cretinism, in its classical form is relatively rare. The lesser degrees are not so rare as we supposed; we simply fail to recognize them. The cases of classical cretinism that I have observed yielded no material for pathologic study, hence they need not be mentioned here. On the other hand, modified cases associated with thyroid enlargement are not uncommon in young persons, and are not infrequently just candidates for the removal of the gland. The improvement these cases show after operation forces our attention to the possibility that the condition may be dependent on some deleterious products of the gland rather than a lack of normal secretion. These cases further suggest that a part of the difficulty is something besides a thyroid minus state, inasmuch as many such cases in late adolescence are not benefited by the use of thyroid extract.

Obviously it is necessary to supplement our clinical observations with a study of the underlying anatomic factors. Fortunately recent developments in thyroid surgery now permit us to secure this material without mental equivocation. First of all we have learned that no secretion is better than that provided by the maldeveloped gland. There is no lack of reported improvement following even a partial removal of the gland. Notwithstanding these salutary results the bogey of too radical operation has prevented surgeons from following this lead.

That myxedema may follow surgical operations has been proclaimed to high heaven since Kocher's studies, made more than fifty years ago, showed that myxedematoid states followed the total removal of the gland in children. His studies, or rather the manner of presenting them, gave surgeons a fright from which they are just beginning to recover. He observed that complete removal of the gland resulted in a state which was called by him "cachexia thyreopriva," that is to say cachectic states resulting from depriving his young patients of their goiters. That it failed to follow total thyroidectomy in adults he did not emphasize.

As noted before, the result of Kocher's studies was that surgeons feared this possibility in patients of all ages and if thyroid deficiency followed operation concluded that too much of the gland had been removed. No one stopped to inquire whether the deficiency appeared because of the operation or in spite of it, or was present even before the operation. This fact cannot be too often repeated nor too strongly emphasized.

Happily the surgical pathologist is now in a position to re-examine this whole problem in the light of the newly acquired knowledge that complete removal of the thyroid gland from adults does not result in notable myxedema. The study of this material has turned up numerous important facts, the chief one being that there is in a broad way a more or less specific myxedema pathology indicating a dysfunction. What is still more important, we are enabled to study what happens when the patient is relieved of the entire gland. This spares us the necessity for speculating on the consequences of removing half of a physiologic disturbance.

Furthermore, the fact that total thyroidectomy can be performed without deleterious consequences compels us to question anew our notions regarding the functions of the thyroid gland in the adult. It suggests the possibility that the functional importance of this organ in the adult has been much exaggerated. Our faith in the usefulness of the thyroid has led us to believe that myxedema is a state in which the thyroid gland ceases to function. Since it has been demonstrated that the adult can get along very well without his thyroid one is compelled to question the possibility of myxedema being due to a deleterious product of a diseased gland. That is to say, instead of a reduced normal secretion, the gland may be producing some substance which is causing the myxedema. It is possible, in other words, that in the myxoid state the thyroid gland does something instead of nothing.

Total removal of the gland enables us to observe what happens when the alleged deleterious products which produce the typical clinical condition are eliminated; it also affords opportunity to study the material obtained from the various incipient stages of the disease. This makes it possible for us, in a measure at least, to anticipate by anatomic study cases which will ultimately present symptoms of a myxoid state.

Predicting the development of postoperative hypothyroidism from a study of the part removed, absolves the surgeon from responsibility of producing what was already on the way. The problem is complicated by the fact that most cases in which a hypo state develops are only temporary, since all evidence of it disappears after some months. These temporary states cannot be predicted from a study of the part removed.

Furthermore, a very radical thyroidectomy results in a number of factors which make it seem probable that the spontaneous myxedematous gland is producing a deleterious something tending to cause the disturbed state. Several substances may be produced in the thyroid gland, myxedema being the state in which the injurious substance is not neutralized. It is known that in myxedema iodine is quickly eliminated from the thyroid gland. We may assume that something has happened which permits this elimination. The study of the histology suggests that the trouble lies in the acinal cells, changes which render a normal function impossible having taken place in them. If one wishes to theorize he can assume that the taking of thyroid extract neutralizes the poisonous substances produced by these cells.

One must hasten to say that in spontaneous myxedemas associated with complete atrophy of the gland these cells are absent and that there seems to be no secretion of any kind.

On the other hand, in those curious cases in which a hyperplastic toxic goiter is in a stage of transition from a hyper to a hypo state we have symptoms of both diseases—both hyperthyroidism and myxedema. Surely one substance cannot be both plus and minus; two processes must be going on simultaneously. I am convinced that the association of the two processes is much more common than is generally supposed. Premyxedematous states may be associated with nervous phenomena which we, ignoring the signs of an impending hypo state, assume are due to a hypersecretion.

If we study a certain type of patient, one thought to be thyrotoxic, yet one sluggish of mind and gaining in weight, some very instructive pathologic pictures are obtained. We call these polyglandular affections —likely they are. Nevertheless, it is also possible that a polyglandular condition may exist in the thyroid itself, as I suggested many years ago. Since this possibility can be studied only in material obtained at operation, it is best to discuss it in the section on postoperative hypothyroidism.

In order to emphasize the importance of studying the lesser hypothyroid states it seems desirable to divide the spontaneous group into the clinical myxedema, those which can be diagnosed by the generally recognized clinical signs, and those in which the picture is recognized as submyxedematoid states, perhaps as premyxedematoid states. The postoperative hypothyroid state falls naturally into groups which are temporary and those which are permanent.

Spontaneous Myxedema
   Clinical Myxedema
   Submyxedematoid States
Postoperative Hypothyroidism
   Postoperative Myxedema
   Temporary Hypothyroidism

SPONTANEOUS MYXEDEMA

Spontaneous myxedema, as noted above, is a clinical condition for which we surgeons can in no wise be held responsible. It was recognized before it was understood—assuming that we understand it now. That is to say, when it was first described we did not know that it was associated with disturbances of the thyroid gland. We are even yet so much occupied with the old classical clinical picture that we have neglected the incipient states. As in all classical clinical cases there is necessarily a stage preceding the full development of the clinical picture. The premyxedematoid states have been very little studied, particularly by surgeons. We still are prone to wait for the basal rate to make the diagnosis for us. This and the use of thyroid extract are depended on to identify the disease. Although some cases attain the early stages of the classical disease there are others which never become typical clinical myxedema; why they do not is just as much a mystery as why atypical hyperthyroid states exist which never develop into typical hyperthyroid pictures.

A more careful study directed toward the early discovery of a hypo state is important to the surgeon because it reveals that in many cases there may be a deficiency which is first recognized after operation. Such a study is facilitated by first considering the typical clinical cases and then the submyxedematoid states separately.

Clinical Myxedema. Classical myxedema shows itself by a thickening of the subcutaneous tissue; it is truly an edema resulting from myxoid changes in the subcutaneous tissues. The chief clinical signs are a mental sluggishness, dry hair and skin, a sensitiveness to cold and a slowing up of all the bodily functions.

Myxedema should be regarded as a final stage of a thyroid disease. Time was when a malodorous vaginal discharge was regarded as an important sign of cancer of the cervix. Full blown myxedema falls in the same category and indicates that we have failed to recognize the early signs.

The underlying anatomic conditions are less easily determined. In general one may say that there are two such conditions: degeneration of the thyroid gland due, first, either to a congenital influence or to secondary changes in colloid goiters; or, second, evolving as the final stages in re-

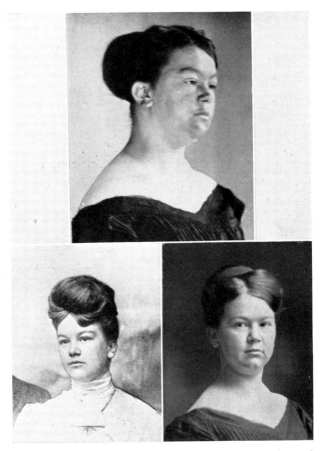

Fig. 177. Extreme case of spontaneous myxedema. Below, the patient 5 years before the onset of the myxedema and the appearance after taking thyroid extract 6 months.

active processes. Both these conditions make it obvious that we should first think of a perverted secretion rather than of a diminished one.

Pathogenesis. Cases which I have been able to observe throughout the years of the development of the disease first show a mental sluggishness. The alert business man becomes indifferent, neglectful, goes broke. He loses his initiative; at first he may note and deplore the fact, but later he becomes irritable when reminded of it. Ideas come slower and he may sit for long periods doing just nothing. He increases in weight, apparently from inactivity, but soon classical signs manifest themselves.

The gain in weight is seen to be due to increase of tissues in certain parts of the body. This is most strikingly apparent in the suprascapular region, where it shows up as heavy pads. The face likewise becomes

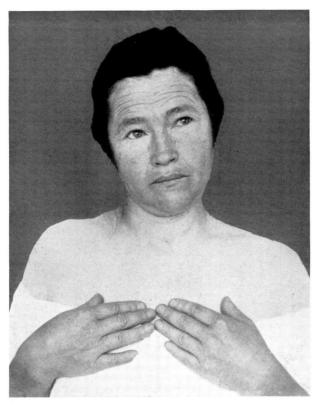

FIG. 178. Myxedema. Age 39, looked much older. Menopause 10 years previous. Eyelids thickened. Forehead wrinkled. Cannot sweat. Mentally very sluggish. Rapid improvement on thyroid extract.

swollen and moonshaped, hence expressionless (Fig. 177). The skin of the forehead buckles into folds, forming transverse ridges. The fingers become thickened and the hands paddle-like so that the patient grows clumsy in handling things (Fig. 178). The feet undergo similar changes, consequently walking becomes awkward and even uncertain. The hair thins out especially round the temples and occiput and for the most part is fine but dry.

Most patients present no such classical picture. They show the increase in weight one usually expects subsequent to the menopause, the age at which this disease is most common. But the typical increase specified in certain regions above mentioned is lacking. Their mental hesitancy may suggest only the tranquillity generally ascribed to advanc-

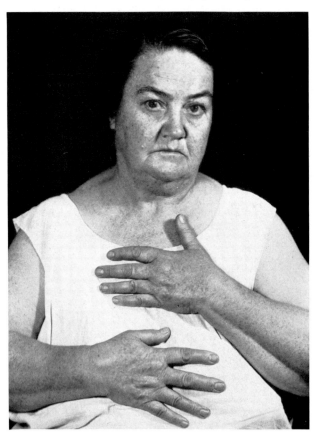

FIG. 179. Spontaneous myxedema. Complacent lady of 54. Lost her hair 8 years ago. Doubled her weight in the last 20 years. Thyroid not palpable. Very sensitive to cold. Fell easily. Was wakeful. All signs cleared on thyroid extract.

ing years (Fig. 179). Others again appear to resent the inquisitiveness of the clinician, showing an irritability which may mask intellectual sluggishness (Fig. 180). The deliberate weighing of the answers, however, reveals the mental sluggishness. A thickening of the lids which causes the patient to look out of slits (Fig. 181) forms part of the picture.

The most common subjective sign is sensitiveness to cold. In times gone by when women wore clothes one could determine whether this sensitiveness existed by counting the layers of their petticoats. Since these garments are no longer worn, so it is said, this valuable clinical sign is lost. Often now the dryness of the skin and hair must be depended upon as clues.

The first sign of a disturbed thyroid function may be not mental sluggishness but mental irritability, spontaneous—without cause and

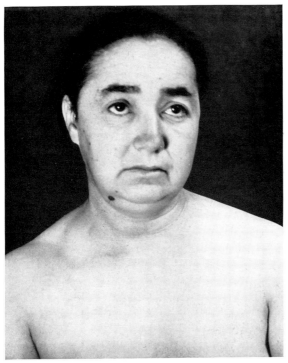

FIG. 180. Myxedema associated with a reserved nervous state. The hair at the temples is thinned. The thickening of the supraclavicular pads is evident.

without any relation to other factors. These early signs are likely to occur at about the menopause and may be ascribed to it. Likewise if the patient is sensitive to temperature changes one ascribes this also to the menopause and the impending myxedema is overlooked. In these cases the basal metabolic rate may not be altered. However, in a nervous patient, in the above sense, with a low rate—30 or less—the possible presence of an impending myxedema should be suspected.

Myxedematous patients do not live out a normal expectancy. Sometimes intercurrent diseases terminate their existence, and sometimes they just spontaneously die without any apparent cause. They become dropsical and albuminuric; their hearts grow irregular, slow; the pulsations are very faint and irregular in rate and volume, in fact there is a typical cardiotoxic state. This is much more likely to occur in cases in which the myxedema develops on a pre-existing goiter. Those attended

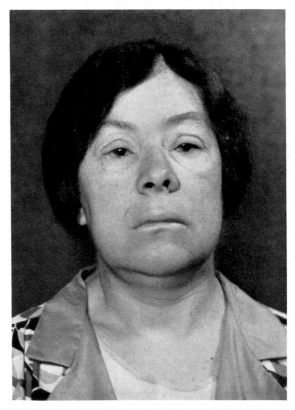

Fig. 181. Spontaneous myxedema. The thickening of the eyelids narrows the palpebral fissure giving a languid expression.

by thyroid atrophy may attain a ripe old age. I have one patient who has been taking thyroid extract for nearly 40 years.

Instead of this gradual development, the symptoms may be initiated by something such as an inflammatory goiter, a nonsuppurative thyroiditis or a Hashimoto's struma (Fig. 182).

Pathology. From the foregoing it is obvious that we must begin the study of myxedema before there are obvious clinical signs. As indicated above a bosselated thyroid in early life or a reactive gland in adults

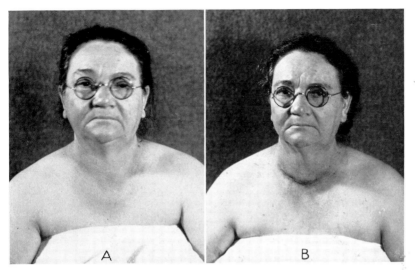

FIG. 182. *A*, Myxedema associated with Hashimoto's goiter. *B*, Spontaneous recovery from the myxedema following a total thyroidectomy.

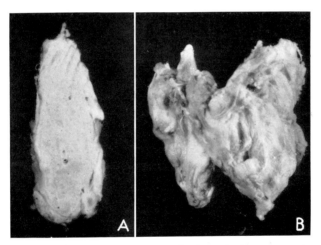

FIG. 183. Thyroids from spontaneous myxedemics. *A*, Autopsy specimen. *B*, Removed by total thyroidectomy.

should suggest that a clinical myxedema is in the offing. A hard goiter which is nontoxic should be regarded at the operating table as a potential postoperative myxedema.

In general, three types of thyroid gland may be distinguished; the atrophic, the adenomatous and the reactive.

The atrophic is so called because the gland is small (*A*, Fig. 183), and seldom palpable in the clinic. On section it is white, apparently entirely fibrous. At the present time only autopsy material and a single specimen obtained by total thyroidectomy (*B*, Fig. 183) have been available for the study of this type.

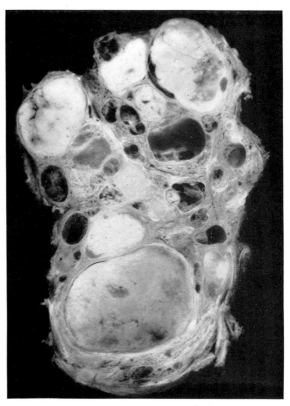

FIG. 184. Cretinoid goiter. Deaf mute, aged 18. Goiter first noted at 3 years of age. Physically of normal size. Gland is made up of miniature nodules fetal in type.

The adenoid type derives its name from the fact that the goiter is nodular and some of the changes occurring therein warrant the use of this term. The entire gland is made up of nodules. In fact many of the nodules are exact counterparts of fetal adenomas (Fig. 184). This is seen in adolescence. It is related to the cretins, the only difference being that development is less retarded. These should be regarded as developmental anomalies rather than as diseased states. Yet it is an anomaly which injures the patient as is shown by his improvement when

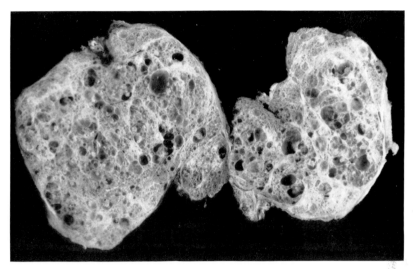

FIG. 185. Cretinoid goiter. Female, age 21. Goiter noted at an early age. Physical characters those of myxedema. Disposition obstreperous. Disposition much improved by a near total thyroidectomy.

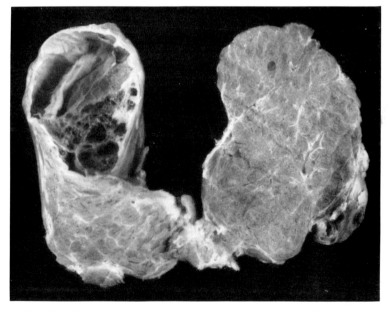

FIG. 186. Gland from a case of myxedema. A cystic nodule occupies the upper pole. The remainder of the gland is simple colloid.

the goiter is removed. Sometimes instead of the goiter being nodular it is cystic, and contains very little thyroid tissue and that little is defective (Fig. 185). These conditions are closely related to the fetal adenomas which are common in adult glands and goiters.

The gland sometimes is cystic and contains papillations which have the same significance here as they do in fetal adenomas. In adults, on the other hand, the greater part of the gland may be normal and only a

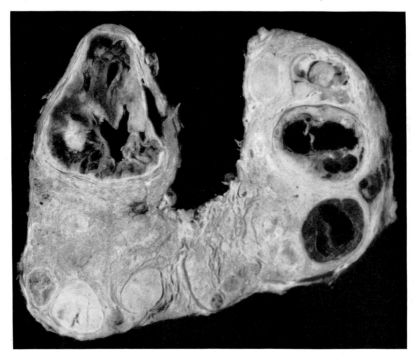

FIG. 187. Cretinoid goiter. F., age 21. Backward as a child but later developed nearly normally. At 15 goiter appeared. Was treated with thyroxin. Bilateral lobectomy followed by partial improvement. Much improved by near total 'ectomy four years later.

single nodule (Fig. 186) be affected. In these the preponderant normal gland should have preserved the patient from myxedema had the generally accepted theories been correct. The degeneration may be secondary, the myxedema appearing after a normal period of adolescence (Fig. 187). In these there must have been a functioning area which later gave way to degeneration.

The reactive type has the physical characters of a thyroiditis; namely, a Hashimoto's goiter. The gland is uniform in outline, hard, grayish white when cut across. It was noted in the chapter on inflammations that this type tends to end in myxedema and, as was above noted, is presumptive evidence of an impending myxedema whether the patient is operated on or not.

Histology. In harmony with the discussion of the gross the histology of the various types may be considered in order.

The fibrotic type, as one might expect, is made up of dense bundles of connective tissue showing little evidence of parenchymatous structure (Fig. 188). Those developing on a pre-existing goiter present a dif-

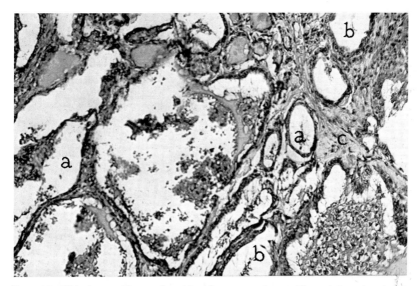

FIG. 188. Slide from a fibrous thyroid without myxedema. The acini are for the most part devoid of epithelium: *a,a,* large acini totally devoid of epithelium; *b,b,* small acini containing an atrophic epithelium; *c,* poorly staining connective tissue. There are no "myxoid" cells.

ferent picture. The low power shows a general fibrosis in which are imprisoned alveoli, many without lumina and all without much colloid (*A*, Fig. 189). The high power shows the acini to be without colloid; the cells have palely staining nuclei; their borders are indistinct; the protoplasm is granular and foamy (Fig. 189). These cells are so frequently found in myxedema that one should suspect a hypothyroid state, present or impending, whenever they are discovered.

In minor myxoid states the interacinal spaces are filled with more deeply staining cells (Fig. 190) while the acinal epithelium is flat and the colloid sparse, palely staining or basophilic.

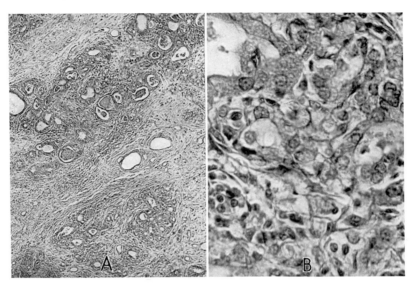

FIG. 189. Atrophic goiter in myxedema. F., age 40. *A*, Heavy bundles of fibrous tissue with few nuclei. The acini contain little colloid. *B*, High power. Large foamy cells with indistinct borders and nuclei. These may be tentatively accepted as myxedema cells.

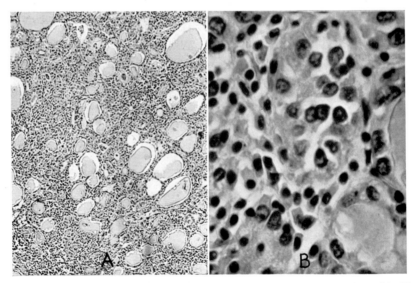

FIG. 190. Moderate myxedema. *A*, The acini contain a small amount of colloid. The cells are atrophic. The interacinal areas contain many cells. *B*, High power. Cells of varying size and stainability, and suggest the "myxoid" type. Acini are partly defective in epithelium.

When implanted on old colloid goiters the epithelium is usually defective, often desquamated (Fig. 191). The connective tissue stains poorly. Large cystic spaces are found, sometimes with papillations which are already evident in the gross, as one sees them in fetal adenomas. The colloid is of varying stainability by special dyes. Much of it refuses any stain. This is the picture in aged myxedemics with old degenerated colloid goiters. This structure is sometimes found in atrophic thyroids that have never been the site of a goiter.

In cases in which myxedema follows Hashimoto's struma, the ana-

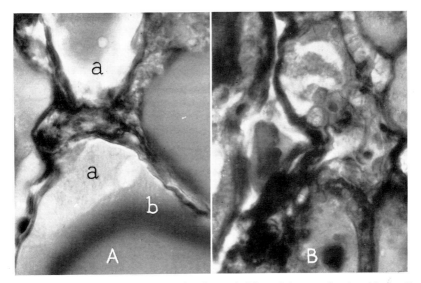

FIG. 191. Slide from a degenerated goiter. *A*, The acini are quite devoid of cells: *a,a*, colloid faintly staining; *b*, more intensely staining with aniline blue. *B*, The epithelium is exfoliated, in large measure degenerated. Some of these cells suggest a "myxoid" state.

tomic changes characteristic of that disease are in evidence. The fibrous bundles are interspersed with many lymphoid cells (*A*, Fig. 192). When the stage of myxedema is reached the acini have usually disappeared (*B*, Fig. 192). The cells are for the most part irregular in size, the acini degenerated (*B*, Fig. 192).

The Submyxedematoid State. Those who have had occasion to observe patients through a long period of years have seen some in whom the myxedema was preceded by conditions not generally recognized as myxedemic. These premyxedematoid stages were referred to in the preceding section.

We have in mind here a series of cases some of which suggested myxedema but never reached a stage where it was recognizable clinically. Others suggested a hypo state only because the condition was ameliorated by the use of thyroid extract. These cases are discussed separately with considerable trepidation. They are poorly defined and become impressive only when studied, together with the anatomy of the gland, over a period of years. These are of great interest to the surgeon because though they are clinically indefinite the anatomic study enables him to recognize their tendency to myxedema which not only indicates that a postopera-

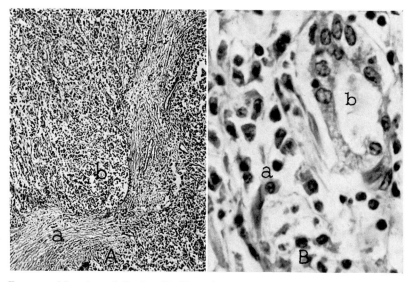

Fig. 192. Myxedema following Hashimoto's struma: *A,a,* bundles of cellular fibrous tissue; *b,* masses of irregular cells; *B,* high power; *a,* interacinal cells irregular in shape and stainability; *b,* acinus with palely staining foamy cells. This picture is that of a Hashimoto's struma.

tive myxedema will develop but that it is already in the offing. Furthermore, it gives evidence that had the operation been more radical a postoperative myxedema would not have developed. The irritation of the operation may augment the pre-existing tendency to myxedema.

Pathogenesis. The early beginning of these cases is such that the possibility of myxedema goes unrecognized and the patients are regarded as thyrotoxic. This supposition is based on the fact that the patient is irritable, has a goiter and that the pulse is rapid. In fact many are preceded by a typical thyrotoxic state. Though they give evidence of a toxic state they are mentally sluggish, and in the privacy of our office we are

apt to think of them as dumb and ornery. A gain in weight and sensitiveness to cold may be the first presentiment that something else portends.

Submyxedema is commonly implanted on the nodular nontoxic
goiter. The irritable state mentioned above is then regarded as a transition to the toxic state and the surgeon operating for that supposed toxic
state finds himself possessed of a patient with postoperative myxedema.
Supposedly toxic states attended by a gain in weight, without a previous
loss, may be the only warning sign.

Curiously enough these patients do not admit they are nervous. One
must quiz husband or friend in their absence to get a true idea of their
nervous condition. If such inquiry reveals an increasing nervousness
which the patient denies, one may be pretty sure something organic is
going on. It is generally agreed by alienists that no crazy person ever
admits his insanity.

The nervous states may be even more subtle. Changes in personality,
lack of interest in things which previously held their attention, particularly when attended by increase in weight and sensitiveness to cold, are
highly suggestive. Sometimes sexual frigidity is the earliest sign. In
many cases the blonde stenographer is blamed when the real cause is a
thyroid disturbance.

The eye of the wise old family doctor will detect many changes in
the personality of a patient who has long been known to him, assuming
that the surgeon is of a too recent vintage to see these things for himself.
Here is where the diagnosis of submyxedema should be made.

Without at any time ever having been toxic these patients are likely
to enter a thyrocardiac state which continues until ended by a typical
cardiac death.

Pathology. The gross pathology may be that of a nontoxic nodular
goiter, usually of long duration, or a uniform one of more recent development. The single suggestive sign is a hard gland without a corresponding
toxic state. In many cases only a small part of one lobe may show this
increase in firmness so that it escapes the palpating finger. These areas
are in fact localized conditions which when general are called Hashimoto's
struma.

On the other hand, the gland may be small, fibrotic and not palpable
in the clinic. This is the type that is most helped by the use of thyroid
extract and that does not tend to a cardiotoxic state.

Histology. As implied above the histologic changes are those of an
incipient chronic lymphoid thyroiditis (Hashimoto's struma). The
earliest stage is represented by an area of lymphoid thyroiditis and by a
group of lymphoid cells which surround the acini (*A*, Fig. 193). At first

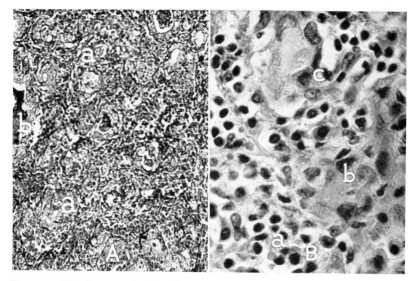

FIG. 193. Slide from a goiter in which at operation no special changes were suspected: *A,a*, lymphoid infiltration; *b*, acinus with low epithelium; *B*, high power; *a*, interacinal cellular masses; *b*, degenerated foamy cells which are the remains of the acinal cells, *c*, acinus with atrophic cells.

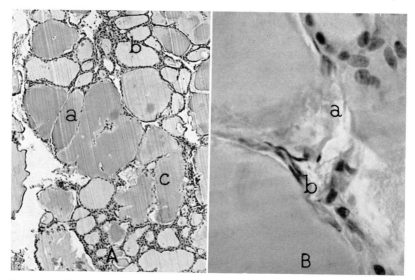

FIG. 194. Slide from a submyxatoid patient: *A,a*, acinal walls indistinct; *b*, colloid thin faintly staining; *c*, colloid basophilic; *B,a*, acinal walls all but destroyed; *b*, epithelium exceedingly atrophic.

the enveloped acini show little change. Later the colloid becomes clumpy, an irregular mass lying in the center of the acinal lumen (*B*, Fig. 193). The acinal cells swell and ultimately fill the entire lumen. These cells are palely staining, even foamy in appearance. Their presence is the most common finding in all myxedemas.

On the other hand, the fibrotic glands may show acinal degeneration marked by complete absence of the cells; even the walls may have disappeared (Fig. 194).

POSTOPERATIVE HYPOTHYROIDISM

By postoperative myxedema is meant a state in which the symptoms follow an operation on the thyroid gland. The surgeon usually assumes it is due to the operation, which, as above noted, may be anything but the truth.

We need to study more in detail, and over a greater length of time, just what takes place after operation. In the preceding section it was emphasized that many patients who are operated on are already the subjects of an incipient hypothyroidism. The symptoms may be exaggerated after operation. When hypo symptoms develop the first thing to do is to study anew the signs and symptoms manifested prior to operation. It is generally believed that the coexistence of hyper and hypo symptoms is rare. I doubt it. Furthermore, when hypo symptoms develop they may be permanent or temporary. Pathologic study suggests that the permanent cases were hypo before the operation. Chesky, of this clinic, has made the important observation that hypo states developing after the resection of degenerated goiters are likely to be permanent while those developing after operations on the acute toxic hyperplastic goiters seldom continue for more than a few months. It is desirable to discuss separately cases in which the myxedema is permanent and those in which the signs of myxedema are incomplete and temporary.

Postoperative Myxedema. Postoperative myxedema in the strict clinical sense is rare. After operation the patient becomes sensitive to cold and develops mental sluggishness; there is a complete picture of clinical myxedema and the patient may feel better when taking thyroid extract. This condition may continue indefinitely. Such cases are true myxedemas which follow operation.

Of course it is possible to operate on incipient myxedemics which become worse after operation, but they are not thereby made postoperative myxedemics as we are wont to assume. I would venture the tentative opinion that if there is permanent myxedema following operation the groundwork was present before operation. There are exceptions, but on the whole we may say that myxedema develops in what we leave behind. The corollary is: don't leave anything to speak of behind.

Pathogenesis. If we assume that a hypo state after operation indicates that too much of the thyroid gland was removed, how are we to account for the fact that when an equal amount of the gland is left in another case a hypo state does not develop? For instance, one of the most pronounced cases of a postoperative hypo state we ever saw in this clinic was that of a woman near the menopause who had a fetal adenoma, the size of a lemon, in the right lobe. This adenoma was removed, leaving the right lobe itself, which seemed normal, practically intact. The left lobe was apparently normal and was not even exposed. After the operation nearly all her thyroid gland remained and was presumably normal, yet a hypo state developed and has continued unchanged. Obviously something must have happened to the structure of that part of the gland left after the operation. In order to solve such a problem we must go to the excised part of the gland, but in this case nothing except a degenerated fetal adenoma had been removed, and that cleanly. Leaving much or little does not protect us against sequence of operation and hypothyroid state.

If one operates on incipient myxedema, in most cases the part of the gland removed shows the structure of the part allowed to remain. This is particularly true in Hashimoto's struma. The acini are interspersed with cells, generally called lymph cells, as has been discussed in the chapter on thyroiditis and in the section on submyxedema. Some surgeons have warned against operating on thyroiditis because postoperative myxedema is likely to develop. The fact is that if one finds he has operated on a goiter showing the anatomic picture of a Hashimoto's thyroiditis he may expect a postoperative hypothyroidism, not because of what he removed but because of what he left. After partial resection of a goiter in a mildly myxedemic patient the development of a hypo state is hastened. The reaction that follows cutting through the crippled gland must be the exciting factor.

If the anatomic changes above noted have anything to do with the production of the hypothydoid state, as they no doubt have, the logical thing to do is a complete thyroidectomy, thus relieving the patient of that part of the gland which would, if left, continue its destructive course and produce a real myxedema. In other words, the myxedema develops because of the unavoidable trauma—not because the operation was too radical but because it was not radical enough.

A thyroiditis is not the only forerunner of myxedema. Instead there may be an atrophic state which is the result of a hyper state. Most likely the patient gives a history of hyperthyroidism in years past, often twenty or more years. Less often both states coexist. The symptoms of a Graves' disease may be present and with it unmistakable evidence of a hypo state. Just because the patient is evidently the victim of a Graves' disease is no reason for assuming that a hypo state is not associated. It is interesting to note in passing that a hypo state following a hyper state does not tolerate thyroid extract. The heart is rendered irregular in rate and volume. In some cases, however, there is nothing in the history or examination which indicates a preliminary hyper state, yet the slide shows evidence of an old hyperplasia. These may confuse the pathologist if he has not been informed of the clinical history.

From the foregoing it is evident that microscopic study of some glands after operation affords no evidence of an approaching hypo state. In these we must assume something happens to the part of the gland allowed to remain. Possibly the operation produces on the remaining part of the gland a reaction comparable to chronic lymphatic thyroiditis (Hashimoto's struma) or at least some traumatic reaction. If this be the case it is something quite different than having removed too much of the gland. This is indicated in the case previously cited in which nearly the whole gland was untouched. As previously regretted, material for the study of this problem is not available. In postoperative myxedemics we should remove that part of the gland which we left behind. Certainly in this clinic the postoperative hypo state has become less common since we started doing very radical operations.

Total thyroidectomies on patients with a spontaneous myxedema have been performed in a very few cases and in only one with an atrophic thyroid. These regularly showed an improvement in the myxedema, consequently further use of thyroid extract was unnecessary. In one case the improvement was so marked that the patient, a spinster of thirty-six, committed matrimony within two years after operation. A number of cretinoid patients have undergone operations, very radical operations, but not complete, with marked improvement. At that time I had not the courage to do a complete removal.

Pathology. The foregoing account of the pathogenesis of the post-operative hypo state in a measure anticipates the pathology. We should be able to tell, goiter in hand, whether or not the patient will show a postoperative hypothyroidism after she recovers from the goiter. We do not know this, but a hard gland suggesting the firmness of a Hashimoto thyroiditis indicates the possibility. If one suspects a postoperative hypo state is likely, the operation should be complete.

The simple negative type does not differ in its gross aspects from other degenerated glands. Sometimes in a degenerated gland (Fig. 195) suggesting the type, seen even in younger persons previously described, a more radical operation is in order.

Histology. A study of excised goiters in which a hypo state followed operation shows a complex picture. The group of intra-acinal cells are characteristic of Hashimoto's struma (Fig. 196). The acini may be crowded, compressed or destroyed, but the characteristic feature is the groups of those cells.

Equally characteristic are cases in which there are a large number of cells in the interacinal spaces but no fibrosis. These are found in areas where the acini are not notably changed.

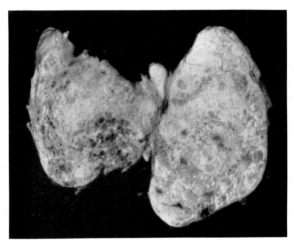

Fig. 195. Submyxedemic goiter presenting hard areas not detected in the clinic but was followed by a postoperative hypo state.

Temporary Hypothyroid State. In many cases a hypo state appears which continues for a time and then disappears. It was noted above that this type is likely to follow operations of hyperplastic toxic goiters. We may assume that some reactive changes take place in the part of the goiter left behind, but that it later recovers. This suggests some sort of postoperative thyroiditis.

Pathogenesis. These temporary hypo states do not reach the clinical dignity of a myxedema. A month or several months subsequent to the operation the patient becomes mentally sluggish, the features become fixed and there may be sensitiveness to cold. The typical padding does not occur and the hands do not become thickened. These states are relieved by the use of thyroid extract. Surgeons are too prone to assume that anything that follows operation must be due to myxedema. Many of these patients fare as well without medication.

Pathology. Generally speaking there is nothing in these glands which suggests a past myxedematoid state at operation or when examined in the laboratory.

Histology. Until we reoperate on these cases after the development of the hypo state we cannot know what goes on in the part of the gland allowed to remain. Since there are no changes suggesting a premyx-

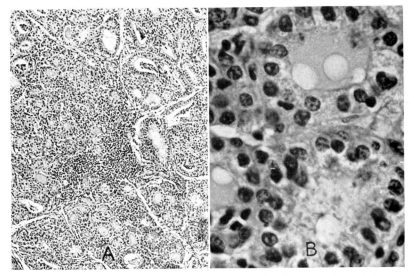

FIG. 196. Slide from a patient who became myxedemic after operation. *A*, The acini are interspersed with a connective tissue infiltrated with lymphoid cells. *B*, The acini show degeneration of the cells. This is in fact the picture of an incipient Hashimoto's struma.

edematoid state in that part of the gland there is no reason to follow the development of this state by a complete thyroidectomy.

Literature

Myxedema. The most important contribution relative to postoperative myxedema was Kocher's (*Arch. f. klin. Chir.*, 1883, 29, 254). In view of the influence this paper has exerted during the last half of the century it is worth while to examine its contents.

He reports 101 cases operated on; of these he deducts 11 operated on during the current year and 13 who died following operation. The remaining 77 he sought to interview. From these 17 were lost track of. Five were cancerous. Of the remaining 55 two more died of intercurrent disease. Of the remaining 53, 34 presented themselves for examination, 19 reported by letter. Those on whom a unilateral operation had been done enjoyed good health, 28 in number. Of those on whom a total operation was done there were 34; of these three died following operation, two died of unknown diseases, and one from cancer. Four of the remainder could not be traced. Of these 18 presented themselves for examination and six reported by letter. Of these six four reported that they were in better health since the operation. Of the remaining two one aged 36 knew no well day following the operation, was sensitive to cold, had loss of sensation in the extremities and a swollen belly. The other, age 38, has been as if paralyzed since the operation. There remain 18 patients on whom total extirpation was done who appeared for examination. One aged 26 recovered and remained well. One aged 12, recovered, feels fine. Of the remaining 16, all complain of some disturbance. Of these 10 are under 20 years of age. Of those older than this two showed marked disturbance: one was 23, the other 45. It is worthy of special note that the 12-year old girl who remained well had a recurrence of her goiter. The clinical sign of cachexia thyreopriva was malaise notably in the extremities, some had actual pain. Sensitiveness to cold comes next. The mental alertness diminished, notably in children still in school. Slowness in speech and in movement was added. Then some swelling of face and extremities. For this condition he selects the name "cachexia strumipriva." Of the two over 20 years, a girl 23 and a man 45, in whom myxedema followed, no further information is available. Thus a case of postoperative myxedema in a man aged 45 has frozen the profession in its tracks for more than 50 years.

Chapter XII

Fetal Adenomas

TO WM. SHAKESPEARE, late of Avon, England, the strangest of all strange things was that men should fear death. To me the strangest thing is that any one should fail to recognize fetal adenomas as independent congenital tumors. They lie imbedded in the normal or diseased thyroid gland, housed in their own capsule, and are as conspicuous as a booze fighter in a Sunday School. They are as distinct from the thyroid gland as the mixed tumors of the salivary glands are from the organs in which they lie. They have the same life history, characterized by slow growth, and their ultimate tendency is to become malignant. So consistently does this hold true that their removal as a prophylactic measure against ultimate malignancy is not only justifiable but mandatory. They do indeed tend to simulate the normal thyroid gland since in middle or late life they usually develop colloid in their follicles, show some evidence of toxicity of degeneration and terminate in a goiter heart. They may, nay must, be regarded as small areas of tissue separated from the thyroid gland early in fetal life and which are enclosed in a separate capsule that boggles their approach to a maturity attained only in later life.

Fetal adenomas frequently are encountered as tiny nodules imbedded in otherwise normal glands. It is inevitable therefore that they should be commonly associated with goiters of all stages. When associated with bosselated goiters they are frequently confounded with the goitrous nodules. Even though associated with goitrous nodules confusion can arise only when both the fetal adenomas and the nodules of colloid goiter are carelessly examined either in the operating room or in the laboratory. In late stages it is true that there may be some confusion, but careful study, gross and microscopic, is sufficient to dispel it.

Fetal adenomas are congenital. In children they are commonly seen as small marble-like nodules quite separate from the remainder of the thyroid gland. They are sometimes associated with the simple colloid goiters of adolescence. This outstanding fact is important clinically: if the goiter regresses these nodules remain, irrespective of whether the disappearance of the goiter occurs spontaneously or coincident with the administration of drugs. Fetal adenomas never regress, they only progress gradually to degeneration, less commonly to malignancy.

237

Though often associated with goiter they quite as often live an existence independent of any other thyroid disease, continuing to expand and displacing the thyroid tissue; when they become large they displace the trachea and may produce pressure symptoms. They tend to grow, that is the important feature to the surgeon. In fact they most certainly will

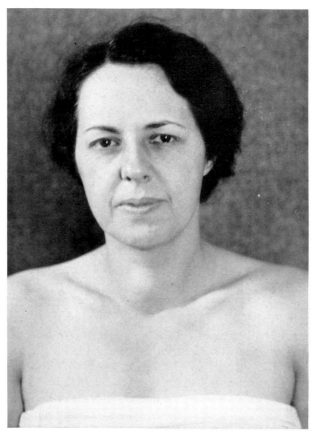

FIG. 197. Fetal adenoma the size of a walnut occupying the right lobe.

grow, consequently no matter how small and insignificant they appear at the moment one can say with assurance that sometime their removal will be imperative because of their size, the toxicity they produce, or, even worse, because of a malignant change they are prone to undergo. One may say with equal assurance that the small nodules in children will cause no serious trouble for a decade or two, so slowly do they grow in early life. For this reason they can be left unmolested for several decades should circumstances make this desirable.

There is one cheerful fact: when fetal adenomas exist independently of diseases of the thyroid proper, their removal cures the patient at once, completely, permanently, and as surely as does the proper removal of a mixed tumor of the parotid.

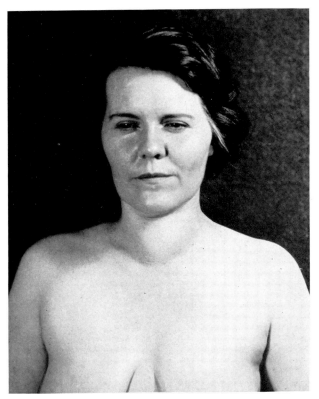

Fig. 198. Multiple fetal adenomas of isthmus and left lobe. Some evidence of toxicity.

Most surgeons and some pathologists refuse to differentiate fetal adenomas from the nodulations of colloid goiters. As above stated the differentiation is nearly always possible in the clinic; certainly in the laboratory. The term "adenoma" has been applied to the nodulations of colloid goiter, perhaps with some justification, as pointed out in the chapter on nontoxic nodular goiter. It should be noted here that if this term is used in connection with colloid nodulations, the prefix "second-ary" should be employed and fetal adenomas should be called "primary adenomas." Though just a compromise, this is better than applying the terms "large follicular adenomas" to the nodules of colloid goiters and "small follicular adenomas" to fetal adenomas.

Multiple fetal adenomas, it may be added here, are frequent concomitants of goiters associated with defective mental development in

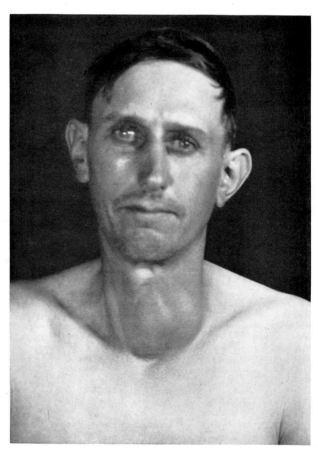

Fɪɢ. 199. Fetal adenoma as large as a goose egg displacing the trachea markedly to the right.

children. In some cases the whole goitrous mass is such an extensive conglomerate of fetal adenomas that there is no thyroid tissue. This betokens that the lesion is congenital and that it is functionally defective.

Pathogenesis. Very small fetal adenomas are sensible only to palpation. In children they can be distinctly felt when they are no larger than a pea. When larger they betray themselves to the eye (Fig. 197), often in the isthmus but quite as often in one or another of the lobes. They may be multiple but this is the exception (Fig. 198). They may be the size of a goose egg or larger (Fig. 199), without presenting any notable symptoms except possibly those due to pressure. But if the patient is carefully observed over a period of years symptoms like those associated with the nodulated colloids will sooner or later be discovered, being due in both instances to the toxicity of degeneration. That is to say, the pulse rate is moderately increased and the patient is somewhat nervous. After the tumor has been removed the patient feels so much better that she expresses surprise at being relieved of something she did not know she had. The advent of toxic symptoms is even more insidious than in colloid goiters.

In their development fetal adenomas may be expected to take one of two directions: develop toxic symptoms as they undergo secondary degeneration, or become malignant. As secondary changes take place, toxic symptoms will develop.

Beginning as they do as small completely encapsulated nodules, the acini of which contain little or no colloid, fetal adenomas usually undergo a belated evolution during which the colloidless follicles in some areas begin to fill with colloid. In late cases a considerable portion of the tumor may be made up of colloid-containing follicles. This is evidence of age rather than portent of size. Tiny nodules no larger than a pea may have almost entirely undergone such changes. But the colloid is never normal and the changes are associated with the development of toxicity. This belated attempt at evolution begins to affect the heart precisely as a degenerating colloid goiter does.

In times gone by I have seen many a cardiac death in cases of only a single fetal adenoma. Nowadays the conspicuousness of the tumor usually leads to its removal before decided cardiac symptoms develop. However the potentiality is there and the early signs are sometimes overlooked even at the present time. The onset is slower and generally comes later in life than that of the degenerated nodular colloids but it will most certainly come sooner or later. Because of the slow development of toxic symptoms without exacerbations and remissions the patient often tolerates them for an astonishing number of years.

When toxic symptoms develop they are progressive, not subject to the remissions and relapses that sometimes occur in colloid goiters; they are never subject to sudden exacerbations; never attain any great height such as one sees in acute toxic goiter; and they are never associated with eye signs. One can assure the patient of these facts when the tumor is small and as yet producing no demonstrable disturbance. However, the toxic symptoms may become very spectacular both as to nervousness and as to loss of weight. Let it be repeated, fetal adenomas never produce exophthalmic goiters. The cysts of fetal adenomas sometimes produce papillary excrescences and these, incredible as it may seem, have been mistaken for the papillations associated with Basedow's disease.

Nor do fetal adenomas produce high degrees of toxicity. There may be considerable irritability, a rapid pulse, and a loss of weight, which, however, is never marked. Apprehension sometimes has more to do with evoking these symptoms than the tumor. This is evident since the symptoms are much augmented when hemorrhages take place in the tumor,— the sudden increase in size, together with some local changes, greatly heightens the previously negligible apprehension.

Almost invariably the mischief caused by fetal adenomas results from secondary changes other than those associated with the growth of the tumor. These changes are regressive and easily differentiated from the secondary evolution above noted. The chief one is the replacement of tissue by cysts. This is possible on such an extensive scale that the entire tumor becomes cystic, only a small margin remaining to proclaim the origin of the cyst. In this way the tumor gradually becomes larger without particularly disturbing the patient until some accident complicates the situation.

The first degenerative changes are noted in the connective tissue, and when this degenerates, it becomes friable and the friability reaches the vessel walls. As a result of this, hemorrhage may take place. These hemorrhages are usually too insignificant to attract the patient's attention, but they can be so extensive that the suddenly increased size of the tumor causes serious compression of the trachea and, if situated substernally, sometimes causes death. In most cases the hemorrhage reaches the capsule of the gland and causes irritation that may be followed by evidence of reaction with edema and tenderness. Sudden pressure due to increase in size of the tumor, or the associated local pain, or both conjointly send the patient scurrying wild-eyed to the surgeon, though the former treated with disdain the latter's warning a few days previous. Opinions as to the capacity of the tumor to cause mischief have suddenly become unanimous.

Lesser hemorrhages may be ignored, especially by the more obtuse patients and those who have never heard of the dire results from a sudden increase in size of neglected goiters.

Low lying adenomas may have escaped the notice of the patient until the hemorrhage occurs. These are usually located behind the sternum.

I have seen sudden dyspnea thus produced that was treated as asthma. The respiratory difficulty however is essentially inspiratory. But when no tumor is palpable and no x-ray available it takes courage to proceed to the removal of such unseen tumors.

With the degeneration of the connective tissue cysts may form gradually. Whether all cysts found in the thyroid gland are secondary to degeneration of fetal adenomas or whether they are primary tumors it is difficult to say. Most cysts contain some adenomatous tissue; and although very small tumors sometimes suddenly enlarge and become painful, as though from hemorrhage, yet it may be only in after years that a simple cyst is removed. Be this as it may, the cystic and solid tumors are closely related in genesis though the capacity of the cysts for belated mischief is confined to hemorrhage and rapid increase in size.

Unimportant but interesting is the tendency of these tumors to undergo calcareous infiltration. Removal is the only salutory thing to do. It is not altogether pleasing when the infiltration involves the surface of the tumor and thereby attaches itself to a large vein and it is even less pleasing when the tumor lies substernally. Hence the careful surgeon will determine the possible presence of such a complication by means of the x-ray before operating. This enables him to distribute his apprehension over a greater period of time and to prepare for eventualities which rarely happen.

Recognition of fetal adenomas at the operating table is important, for they do not involve the thyroid gland proper and their enucleation is all that is required if the gland is not goitrous. Of course when complicating a colloid goiter, as they frequently do, removal of the goitrous lesion is also necessary. It may be noted that the timid operator too often is content to remove the fetal adenoma without determining the state of the thyroid gland. The presence of a fetal adenoma does not preclude the existence of a goiter.

The least common but most important of the changes which fetal adenomas undergo is the development of malignancy. This phase is discussed in the chapter on tumors (XIII). It need only be mentioned here that the small empty acini may proliferate, and, without producing colloid, form elongated columns. The cells proceed to produce their kind without attempting to perform any useful function. When this growth tendency is manifest, there exists a malignant potential which is usually diagnosed as such by pathologists. But the surgeon has the satisfaction of knowing that as long as the new growth is confined to the capsule it is clinically benign; he should not be too sure of it, however, for it may invade a vein before it ruptures its capsule. Metastases may be present when the capsule is apparently intact. Therefore the surgeon should not believe all the pathologist tells him, although it pays to listen.

Pathology. The study of the pathology of fetal adenomas must needs begin with the observation of them in children in the clinic. Here one seldom finds them complicated by other thyroid changes. One can

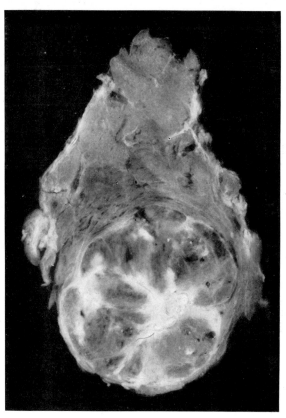

Fig. 200. A fully developed fetal adenoma in an early uniform nontoxic goiter.

feel them, when situated in the isthmus, no larger than a pea, exquisitely encapsulated, perfectly spheroid, hard and shot-like. It is impossible to mistake them for any other lesion. I have observed the gradual growth of these lesions in a number of cases, literally for decades.

When they are associated with general thyroid enlargement one misses these fundamental characteristics, and when associated with nodular goiter they may even engender uncertainty in the clinic as to their identity.

If the thyroid strives to emulate the fetal adenoma and produces rounded tumors, the picture is much confused, as above noted; but even then one can identify the fetal adenomas because they tend to protrude from the goiter proper and form more isolated nodules. Of course when the fetal adenoma is imbedded within the thyroid gland, as is frequently the case when it is small, it cannot be recognized since it is not accessible

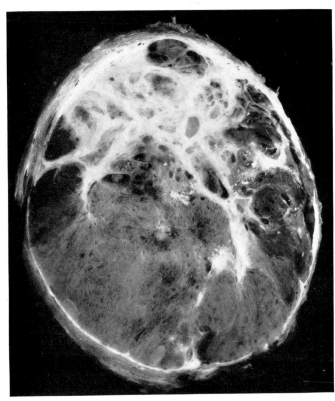

FIG. 201. Degenerating fetal adenoma. The fibrous tissue occupies the upper pole. Below are large cyst-like acini.

to direct palpation. Thus its discovery comes as a surprise when revealed by cutting across a goiter of any kind.

The pathology of the operating table is enlightening. The rounded tumor is encapsulated and is readily removed from the thyroid gland without disturbing that organ. One removes the tumor just as one shells out a lipoma. The characteristic feature in the gross is the ovoid outline of the tumor when exposed at operation. The surface is smooth, lying immediately below the capsule, and it protrudes from the normal gland or above the goitrous gland, if one be present.

The early fetal adenomas appear as uniformly deep red nodules in an otherwise normal gland (Fig. 200). The earliest secondary change is the formation of a stellate fibrous core (Fig. 200). The fibrous tissue in typical cases divides the tumor into lobules like the septa of a grapefruit (Fig. 200). The fibrous area may occupy one pole of the gland (Fig. 201). Sometimes, when several tumors are present, one may show chiefly

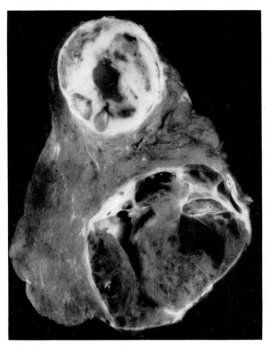

FIG. 202. Multiple fetal adenomas, the upper fibrous, the lower chiefly cystic, the gland otherwise normal.

fibrous tissue while another is formed by large acini and cysts of varying sizes (Fig. 202).

Should the tumor be coincident with a bosselated goiter, the cystic changes associated with the distinct and heavy capsule of the fetal adenoma can always be recognized at the operating table.

However, nodular goiters develop capsules, though they are not as distinct as those of the fetal adenomas (Fig. 203) because the former are produced by compression of parenchymatous tissue of the gland and not primarily by fibrous tissue, as are the latter. Yet when bosselations

of nodular goiters undergo degenerations with liquefactions they resemble quite closely the secondary changes in the fetal adenomas (Fig.
203). In such cases a microscopic study may be necessary to differ-

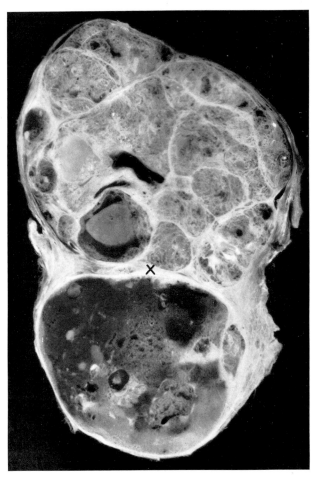

Fig. 203. Nodular goiter associated with fetal adenoma. The nodular part has undergone various degrees of cystic degeneration. The fetal adenoma (below) is in a more
advanced degree of degeneration. The chief distinguishing feature lies in the capsule,
x, which separates the two areas.

entiate them. One may say in general, however, that if the tumor is not
distinctly a fetal adenoma, it is a colloid nodule. The heavy capsule, or
the characteristic fibrous core, usually can be found and either is typical
of a fetal adenoma (Fig. 204). Distinct cysts with thick walls are char-

acteristic of fetal adenoma origin. Such cysts nearly always retain areas of gland structure which bear the distinctive features of a fetal adenoma (*x*, Fig. 205).

Next to the development of malignancy the most important degenerative change is hemorrhage. As previously mentioned, hemorrhage into a cystic area may produce sudden suffocation, especially if the tumor

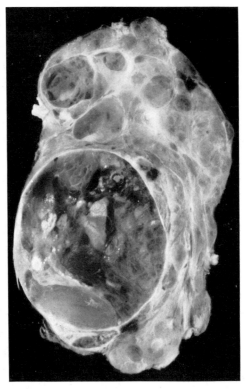

FIG. 204. A fetal adenoma, below, is associated with a colloid goiter. The fetal adenoma has a more distinct capsule than the goiter nodule and areas of degenerated fibrous tissue septa may be noted.

lies beneath the upper part of the sternum. The size of the tumor may be doubled within a few hours, necessitating an emergency operation. Hemorrhage may be so extravagant (Fig. 206) that is produces a fresh clot as large as a teacup.

The tendency of nodular goiters to assume the appearance of fetal adenomas and that of fetal adenomas themselves to develop some adult follicles and become toxic, lies in the fact that both are developed in the same anlage. The difference is that the fetal adenoma is enclosed in a cellophane capsule at a very immature stage, and this isolation prevents its growing apace as the gland develops. The bosselations of nodular goiters develop as a secondary process in the walls of the acini or from fetal rests in the interacinal spaces. That there will be some resemblance in the final stage is obvious, but it is no excuse for not recognizing their genesis and tendency.

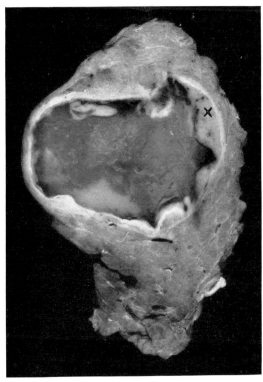

FIG. 205. Thick walled cyst with areas of gland tissue, *x*. Characteristic of origin from a fetal adenoma.

An apparently large uniform goiter may, on section, show a part of the bulk to be made up of a fetal adenoma around which are the nodulations of a colloid goiter. Such curious specimens show how closely the nodulations of goiters are related to fetal adenomas and that though distinct as a whole there is a suffused border-line. A correct conception regarding the genesis of the nodulations of goiter is necessary to appreciate the relationship. These border-line cases do not lend themselves to abstract consideration. They must be studied individually and in detail.

Histology. There are three things which are the distinctive features of the microscopic structure of fetal adenomas; the capsule, the acinal cells and the fibrous septa.

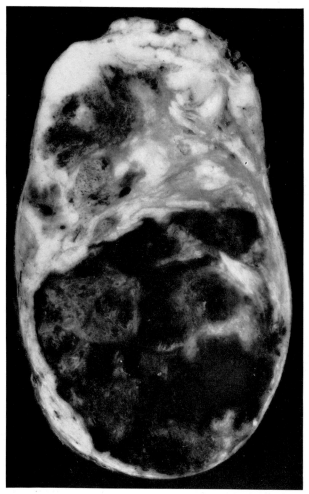

Fig. 206. Large hemorrhage in a cystic fetal adenoma. Below is a large space occupied by a fresh blood clot. Just above is an area of blood-infiltrated tumor. At the top is a margin of active cell proliferation, cancer bound.

The fibrous capsule is best studied by making sections across the tumor, including a part of the fetal adenoma on one side and a part of a goiter on the other (Fig. 207). It is made up of dense layers of fibrous tissue.

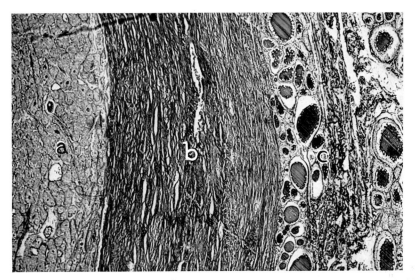

Fig. 207. Capsule of a fetal adenoma including a part of it and a part of the colloid goiter: *a*, fetal adenoma; *b*, the capsule showing heavy bundles of fibers with few nuclei; *c*, compressed area of colloid goiter, in certain areas of which the acini are almost wholly obliterated.

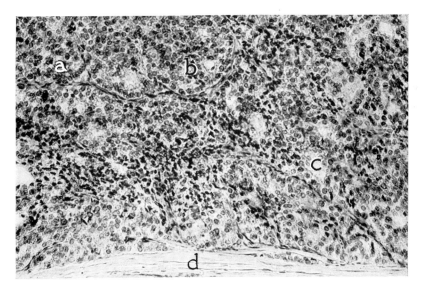

Fig. 208. Slide from a fetal adenoma made up of small acini: *a*, cell masses not defined as acini; *b*, acini without lumina; *c*, acini containing a small amount of colloid; *d*, small section of the capsule, made up of dense fibrous tissue.

Characteristic of the microscopic structure of fetal adenomas are the small acini which have tiny lumina and contain no colloid (Fig. 208). In other words, the structure is that of the normal thyroid approximating the midperiod of gestation. One never sees this picture in any kind of goiter; it is exclusively that of a fetal adenoma.

Sooner or later some of the follicles develop colloid and come to look like regular follicles of the gland in a newborn (Fig. 209). For the most part the development is abortive, the follicles remain small and the colloid they contain stains atypically.

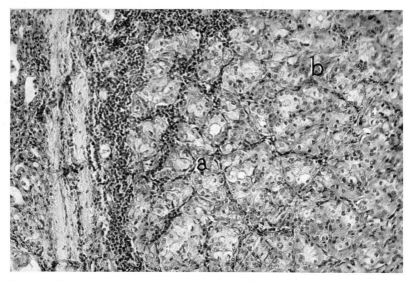

FIG. 209. Beginning follicle formation in a fetal adenoma: *a*, small acini with distinct walls; *b*, fibrous septum; solid cell columns without lumina but with distinctly staining cells preparatory to the formation of lumina. The nuclei are proportionately smaller than in normal thyroids.

With further development the acini become larger and approximate the structure of the acini of colloid goiter, but the colloid they contain is never normal, being thick, thin or granular (Fig. 210). The cells lining these follicles are small, deeply staining and withal like those in the fetal gland. The cells lining the colloid-containing follicles are flat, obviously incapable of forming normal colloid. Such areas viewed alone could not be distinguished from those of colloid goiter were it not that they are always associated with areas of small follicles which exist only in fetal adenomas. Besides there is the distinctive fibrous capsule which is utterly unlike the one made up of compressed acini which form the pseudo-capsule of the nodulations of nodular colloid goiter.

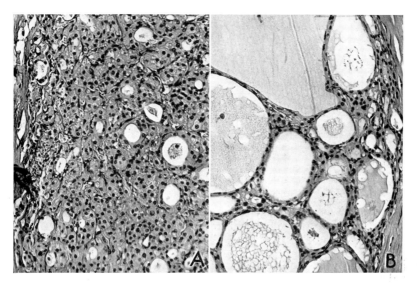

FIG. 210. Fetal adenoma making an abortive attempt to develop normal follicles: *A*, fetal adenoma with small follicles; *B*, larger follicles with flat deeply staining nuclei. The colloid presents various abnormal states, some clear faintly staining, some stainless, some vacuolated, anything but normal.

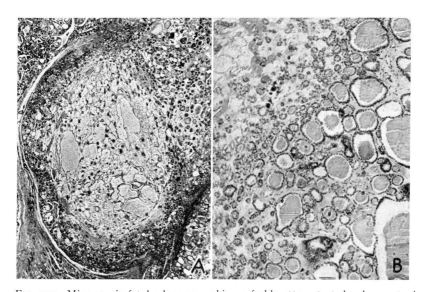

FIG. 211. Microscopic fetal adenoma making a feeble attempt at development: *A*, the nodule in the center shows large cystic acini; *B*, higher power of same showing degeneration as well as imperfect follicle formation. In the upper right the acini as well as the connective tissue have undergone degeneration.

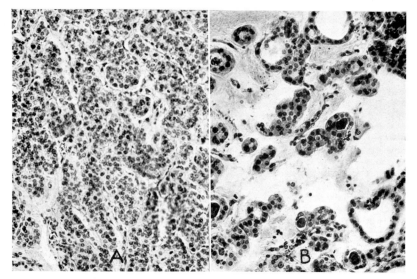

FIG. 212. Fetal adenoma developing solid columns instead of acini: *A*, solid columns arranged more or less in parallel columns; *B*, isolated columns and acini lying in partly liquid connective tissue. As in all fetal adenomas the nuclei are all small and deeply staining.

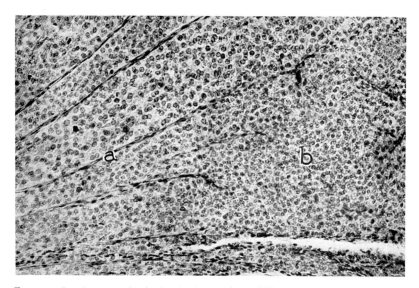

FIG. 213. Lawless growth of a fetal adenoma but still intracapsular: *a*, cells arranged in columns divided by connective tissue septa but without attempt at the formation of lumina; *b*, areas of cells without column formation, and likewise without nest formation.

Microscopic fetal adenomas often show the entire process within a single field of the microscope (*A*, Fig. 211). One may see large cystic acini, areas of connective tissue in process of degeneration and feeble acini with imperfect colloid. The small nodules naturally are accidental findings in otherwise normal glands or in goitrous ones. These secondary changes indicate age, irrespective of the size of the tumor.

The acinal epithelium instead of developing colloid sometimes multiplies and forms cell columns without a lumen. These may be solid columns, closely packed (*A*, Fig. 212), or they may lie more or less isolated in con-

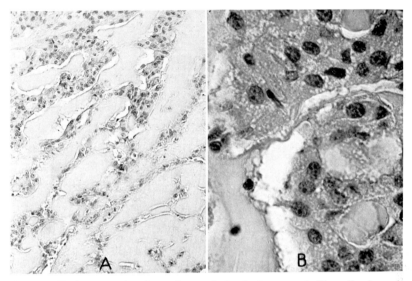

Fig. 214. Early connective tissue changes in fetal adenoma. *A*, The cell columns are compressed by swollen and degenerated connective tissue. *B*, The cells are degenerated, vacuolated and liquefied. In some areas there is beginning liquefaction. The sparse colloid takes the stain indefinitely.

nective tissue which has undergone a high degree of degeneration (*B*, Fig. 212). Such changes represent the first step tending toward malignancy. During the closer approach to malignancy the cell columns increasingly deviate from the normal structure (Fig. 213). In these the cells form irregular columnar masses or may lose all semblance of acinal structure (Fig. 213). They are microscopically malignant though most of them are within the capsule and consequently clinically benign. The same structure is found in those which have escaped the capsule or invaded a vein, and are therefore malignant. These changes will be further discussed in the chapter on malignant tumors (XIII).

The degenerative changes in the connective tissue begin in the septa,

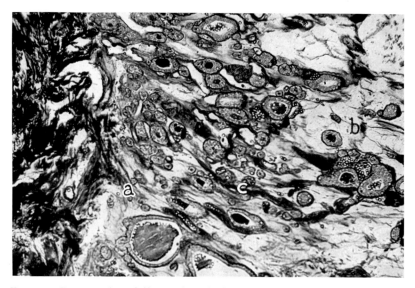

FIG. 215   Degeneration of fibrous tissue in fetal adenoma: *a*, well-staining fibers; *b*, the fibers have lost all affinities for dyes and are in a process of liquefaction; *c*, the acinal epithelium is but faintly staining, in some areas atrophied leaving only a few cells.

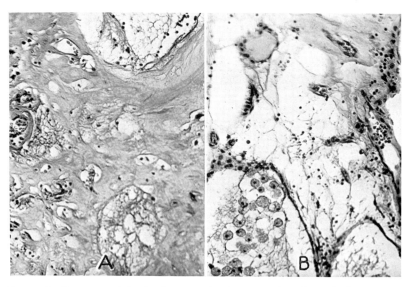

FIG. 216. Degenerated fetal adenoma: *A*, the connective tissue is homogeneous; imbedded in it are small groups of cells—identifiable acini; *B*, all structure is lost and the tissue is gelatinous. Here and there are degenerating nuclei of what were once acini.

which become thick, palely staining or which form indefinite masses not susceptible to any dye (Fig. 214). These may undergo additional degeneration and liquefy (Fig. 215). Within this degenerated mass acini appear as mere shadows of their former selves, the cells being small and palely staining.

In a further stage the degenerative process is even more complete. The acini are marked by small groups of cells (*A*, Fig. 216) lying in a homogeneous gelatinoid mass. In the final change all structure is lost for large areas. Only here and there are acini identifiable (*B*, Fig. 216).

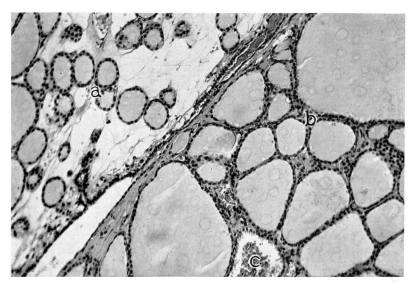

FIG. 217. Small island of fetal adenoma in a colloid goiter: *a*, area of fetal adenoma showing a myxoid stainless connective tissue; the acinal epithelial cells are low with small deeply staining epithelium; *b*, area of simple colloid goiter; *c*, acinus with degenerated colloid.

Any of the structures just described is sufficient to identify the tissue as that of a fetal adenoma. However, small ones like the above are sometimes found in small areas that escape the naked eye, lying between nodules of a colloid goiter (Fig. 217). Occasionally these areas are so small that they occupy only the spaces between adjacent acini. This is of theoretical interest because it may be a link between the still earlier embryonal stage and the interacinar groups of cells.

Literature

Fetal Adenomas. I am under the embarrassing necessity of quoting Hertzler (*Arch. Surg.*, June 1928, 16, 1187–1200) as presenting the clearest exposition of this really simple tumor.

CHAPTER XIII

Tumors of the Thyroid Gland

TUMORS of the thyroid gland hold very little interest for the student of thyroid pathology. For the most part they are just a chapter in the broad field of oncology. However, their relationship to goiters is such that their beginnings are important for, as in all malignant tumors, cure depends on early recognition. This is doubly important in thyroid malignancies because a considerable proportion of them develop on fetal adenomas. The long benign course of these tumors makes them ideal objects for prophylactic removal. Even in cases in which the malignant stage has been reached the slow development makes it possible to cure many of them. On the other hand, those which grow diffusely in a goitrous or in a previously normal gland usually are incurable when the diagnosis is made.

The vast majority of thyroid malignancies are of epithelial origin. Two general types which are widely contrasting must be recognized; those developing in a fetal adenoma as above noted, and those developing diffusely in the goitrous or normal gland.

As previously explained the fetal adenomas form the basis of the majority of malignancies, but in order to harmonize the histologic changes with the clinical behavior one must appreciate their individual peculiarities. In the diagnosis of malignancy superimposed on fetal adenomas the conclusion of the pathologist is often misleading to the surgeon. The broad interpretation in the laboratory includes as malignant, cases that are clinically benign. In order to emphasize this form, not all too sharply defined, I have called them "mixed tumors" because of their similarity both anatomically and clinically to the mixed tumors of the parotid. Therefore the operating room diagnosis must be taken in conjunction with the anatomic study in making postoperative prognosis. A tumor, even though histologically malignant, if confined to the capsule of the tumor, is likely to be clinically benign if there is little metaplasia of the cells. In some cases metastases occur before the capsule is invaded, but at the worst such occurrences are rare.

It is desirable to determine by anatomic study just what the degree of malignancy in the individual case may be so that the efficacy of any treatment can be properly evaluated. The cure of things that were not present has caused so much muddling of statistics that the need of caution, for the benefit of the surgeon, in this matter needs to be emphasized. For instance, if such a premalignant tumor is treated postoperatively by radiation and recurrence does not take place, the use of this agent may be disappointing in cases that are actually clinically malignant.

As in all cancer, the criteria of malignancy are invasion and metastasis. In their absence a diagnosis of thyroid cancer demands careful consideration, particularly in cases of cures. In the absence of these criteria the most careful reconsideration is demanded lest one report as cured, malignancies that never existed. This caution is especially necessary now that radiation so commonly follows removal of tumors the diagnosis of which has not been fully established.

Carcinomas arising diffusely are always very malignant, in fact I have yet to see a cure.

Other malignant tumors are rare. Some pathologists even deny the occurrence of sarcomas. However, diffuse spindleform or round cell tumors which metastasize by way of the blood vessels fit so well into the surgeon's conception of sarcoma that one may be excused if he clings to this diagnosis in such cases. At the same time, tumors develop within the confines of the capsule of a fetal adenoma, hence they are of almost certain epithelial origin, but they may be confusingly spindleform so that the whole course of the disease must be considered in arriving at a final diagnosis.

Benign tumors of the thyroid gland are so rare that they are of little surgical interest.

The tumors of the thyroid gland may as a matter of clinical convenience be classified as follows:

    I. Carcinoma Developed on Fetal Adenoma
   II. Carcinoma Developed Directly on the Thyroid Gland or a Pre-existing Goiter
 III. Mixed Tumors of the Thyroid Gland
 IV. Sarcoma of the Thyroid Gland

This classification does not recognize the existence of metastatic tumors of the gland. The reports of such cases are not convincing. I have not encountered any.

CARCINOMA DEVELOPED ON FETAL ADENOMAS

This is by all odds the most common form of malignant tumor affecting the thyroid gland. Most statistics show the proportion is 80 per cent. This accords with my experience in the clinic. If microscopic diagnosis is made the basis of calculation the proportion is even higher.

I have separated from the general group those in which, though they present cell proliferation, the growth is slow and but little malignant.

Pathogenesis. Fetal adenomas, as set forth in the preceding chapter, usually exist many decades as benign tumors. The approach to malignancy is generally signalized by rapid growth and by increasing hardness. However, since hemorrhage into these tumors is a very common accident, rapid increase in size and density should be considered with caution. The density of malignancy is something different from the elastic hardness of hemorrhage and inflammation of the capsule. The definite clinical evidence of malignancy is escape of the new growth from the tumor capsule and the direct invasion of the tissues of the neck. The area of malignancy may involve only a small part of the tumor and when this lies away from the palpable surface a clinical diagnosis is impossible.

Early the hard gland, before there is invasion of the surrounding tissue, may cause discomfort because of the hardness. The development of a malignancy in a fetal adenoma lacks the rapidity of a hemorrhage. Furthermore in a tumor which from its size alone does not seem large enough to cause direct pressure, but is accompanied by marked discomfort or compression of the trachea, malignancy is likely. When the capsule is being invaded attachment to the adjacent tissue always causes marked pain and disturbance of respiration and often of deglutition if the invasion occurs on the medial surface. If the front or lateral part of the tumor is involved in the new growth, and the adjacent muscle is invaded and the nodules are directly exposed to palpation, recognition of malignancy is easy.

Invasion and compression of the trachea usually is the process that kills the patient. Hemorrhage into a degenerated tumor may cause sudden suffocation by compressing the trachea. Metastases to the lungs and bones and the intestinal tract are the most common sites. I have seen intestinal obstruction due to tumor metastasis as the primary lesion before any disease of the thyroid gland was recognized.

In the fungating form ulcerating lesions may bleed and cause death by the loss of blood. Infection may play a part. If the esophagus is invaded infection may extend to the mediastinum. Or the mediastinum may be extensively invaded by continuity from a low-lying primary tumor. In such cases if there is an absence of a neck tumor, confusion of diagnosis may result. X-ray examination may disclose a tumor of the mediastinum.

Pathology. If a fetal adenoma is hard on clinical examination malignancy must be suspected. Increased density is more impressive at the operating table. Often, once the tumor is exposed, nodulations are per-

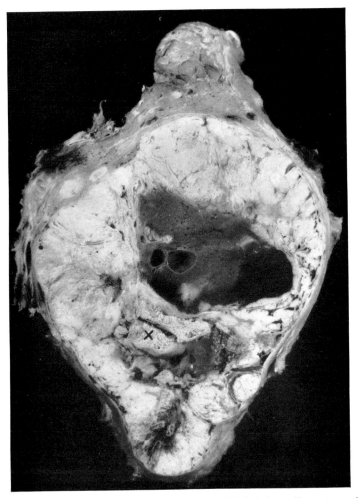

FIG. 218. Fetal adenoma histologically malignant. Definitely malignant at *x*, but the entire upper part of the tumor shows proliferation. Hence histologically malignant but it proved to be clinically benign. Had myxedema which disappeared after operation.

ceived which could not be detected in the clinic. These changes are sufficient to warrant the diagnosis of malignancy. Such tumors, instead of being of a red color like the benign fetal adenoma, are white. Once the surrounding tissue is invaded the diagnosis is simple, but if the invasion of the capsule occurs in some part of the tumor not accessible to palpation it cannot be detected until the operation proceeds.

When the tumor is removed it is whitish, at least that part which is involved in malignant changes, and has the hardness of cancer. The small low nodulations of malignancy are commonly present and give unmistakable evidence of malignancy.

Areas histologically malignant may be found which are so deeply situated that they are not in evidence even at the operating table and are first discovered in the laboratory after the tumor is cut across. Though these are histologically malignant, recurrence does not take place as a rule. However, such cases need to be studied with care because areas elsewhere may show positive evidence of malignancy (Fig. 218).

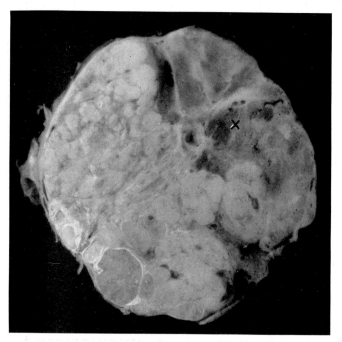

Fig. 219. Carcinoma in a fetal adenoma. All but the area, *x*, is malignant.

Two types may be distinguished on cross-section, those showing gradual invasion through more or less of the gland, and the papillary which develop in a pre-existing cyst.

Usually a considerable part of the tumor shows malignant change but some areas generally retain the fetal adenoma structure (Fig. 219) so that the nature of the tumor is certain. The presence of hemorrhage in malignant tumors usually means that a fetal adenoma was the site of beginning. Such tumors occasionally show nodulations as though several areas had simultaneously become malignant (Fig. 220). Sometimes the cellular invasion is more diffuse. In these cases some areas may be made up of spindle cells giving the general appearance of sarcoma but they invade the capsule like an epithelial tumor and no doubt are such (Fig. 221). Moreover there usually are some areas which make it possible to identify the source of origin of the tumor.

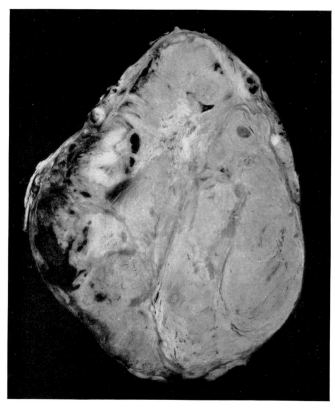

FIG. 220. Malignant fetal adenoma. The tumor is made up of many individual nodules apparently more or less separate.

Those which develop a papillary structure may produce a degenerating fungiform mass filling a previously existing cavity (Fig. 222). The tumor mass is friable and consequently it is easily removed with a finger. In such cases there probably will be a point of invasion of the capsule which is not at once recognizable. In some cases the degeneration obviously preceded the development of malignancy. The greater part is formed by degenerating fetal adenoma with small areas of malignancy (Fig. 223). The existence of a fetal adenoma does not preclude the development of malignancy in the thyroid beyond the fetal adenoma (*x*, Fig. 223). Such incidences should be suspected if the clinical signs are more pronounced than the changes in the fetal adenoma indicate. It is not uncommon to find a fetal adenoma acting as innocent sentinel for a deeply lying diffuse malignancy.

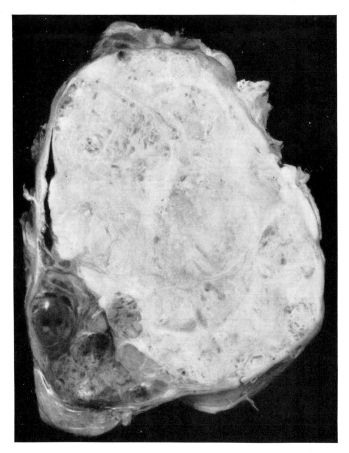

FIG. 221. Malignancy developed on a fetal adenoma. In some areas the growth was diffuse and gave the microscopic picture of a spindle-celled sarcoma.

The papillary formation may be of more vigorous growth and invade not only the capsule of the tumor but the adjacent muscle and skin. These may form bleeding fungiform tumors of huge size. The papillary formation may even be retained in the recurrence (Fig. 224).

Histology. The earliest evidence of tendency toward malignancy is the formation of long columns of cells. This is sufficient to warrant the microscopic diagnosis of malignancy. Diffuse invasion of deeply staining cells is even more distinctive (*A*, Fig. 225). In some tumors the cells are large, palely staining and may show polymorphism in some areas (*B*, Fig. 225). Variation in size and stainability indicates a malignant stage whether the capsule is invaded or not. Some pathologists describe the invasion of blood vessels by cells as the first evidence of malignancy. Either I have not encountered this or its detection transcends my cyto-

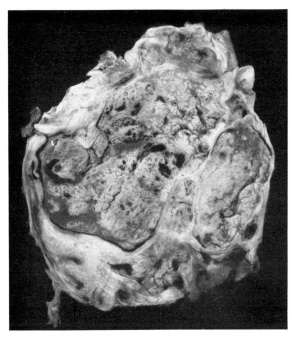

FIG. 222. Fungiform carcinoma developing in a cystic fetal adenoma. The tumor mass was friable and in part hemorrhagic.

logic acumen. That such early invasion does occur is made evident by the occurrence of metastasis before attention is called to beginning malignancy by changes in the tumor.

In some cases solid masses of cells form the tumor. These are irregular in size and stainability and may be spindleform, strongly resembling sarcoma but areas indicating their origin from epithelium stamp them as carcinomas (Fig. 226). This is the type most likely to be attended by distant metastases. Limited fields suggest sarcoma but the study of the entire slide shows areas of transition from typical fetal adenoma acini.

Of particular interest are those cases in fetal adenomas in which the columnar arrangement of the cells bears a very close resemblance to the adrenal cortex (*A*, Fig. 227). Likewise, large foamy cells which very much resemble adrenal tumors (*B*, Fig. 227) are of interest chiefly because these tumors are recorded as being evidence of metastasis in the

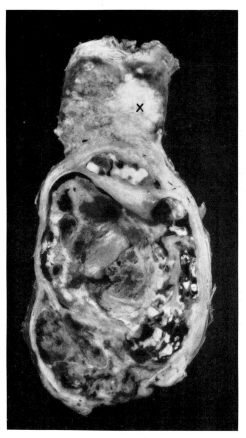

Fig. 223. Malignancy in a degenerated fetal adenoma. The malignancy was confined to a small area in the center of the mass. A second malignancy lies at *x* above the fetal adenoma. It was this part of the tumor that produced the invasion.

thyroid of adrenal tumors. Before such a diagnosis is justified one must either demonstrate the presence of a primary tumor in the kidney or have the patient die of it at some future date.

Malignancy Developed from the Normal or Goitrous Gland. In these cases there is no pre-existing benign tumor. The tumor begins at a certain point, invades the gland and ultimately the surrounding tissues of the neck. It is sometimes difficult in late cases to tell whether the tumor began in a small central fetal adenoma, diffusely in an old goiter, or in a thyroid gland not previously goitrous. If there is extensive invasion throughout the gland, and a portion of it is intact without there being anywhere a demonstrable part of the capsule of a fetal adenoma, it most likely began diffusely. These likewise have the structure of a simple carcinoma whereas those developing in a fetal adenoma present some-

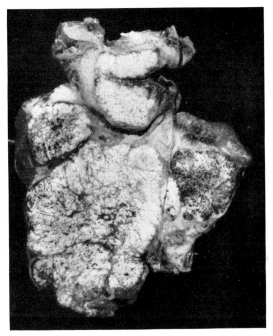

FIG. 224. Papillary recurrence after the removal of a like tumor which had developed in a fetal adenoma.

where histologic evidence of such origin. Often too when there is a cancer on one side, and the other lobe is normal one may assume that the malignancy developed in a thyroid not previously goitrous.

Pathogenesis. The time when these malignancies began cannot be determined. Pain and disturbances of deglutition are usually the first clinical evidence. When a goiter, previously tolerated without local complaint, begins gradually to cause local pain and disturbance of respiration or deglutition, malignancy must be suspected even though no suspicious area can be palpated.

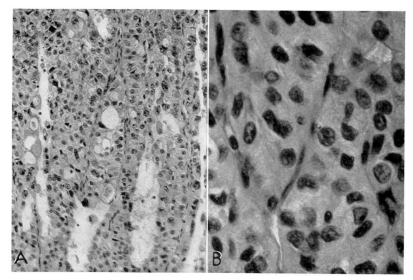

FIG. 225. Early malignant fetal adenoma. *A*, Long columns of cells with many different forms and sizes of cells. *B*, later stage in which the columnar formation is lost save for here and there a spindle cell. The amount of protoplasm is large without any distinct cell borders.

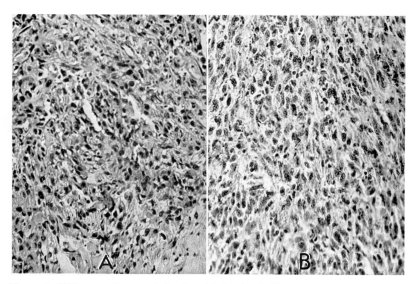

FIG. 226. Diffuse carcinoma of the thyroid gland. *A*, The spheroidal arrangement is for the most part lost. The cells are irregular in size. The cells are in close contact with the vessel walls. *B*, The cells are diffuse and vary much in size and stainability. Some are in a state of degeneration.

Usually a hard mass is detected which at once suggests malignancy. If the site of invasion is medial or backward these disturbances may be quite pronounced before there is palpatory evidence of malignancy or even of a goiter. If the invasion is anterior the low hard nodulations are usually palpable and this is sufficient to determine the nature of the trouble. Of course when the adjacent tissues of the neck are invaded the nature of the trouble is evident enough. Despite every care malignancies may be discovered during the operations which were not detected during the clinical examinations.

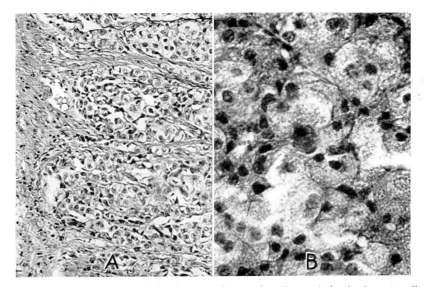

FIG. 227. Structures resembling hypernephromas in goiters: *A*, fetal adenoma cells arranged in columns simulating adrenal cortex; *B*, cells which resemble the foamy cells of a hypernephroma.

Pathology. The evidence outlined above is made more significant as the lesion is exposed at the operating table, when the nodulations and the hardness are revealed. However, not all hard goiters are malignant. Riedel's and Hashimoto's strumas may be exceedingly dense yet there is withal a certain elasticity which is distinctive of a reactive process. But the cross-section may be required to distinguish them. The granular nature of the surface, together with the difference in feel as the knife severs the tissue, is distinctive. The sensation transmitted to the hand as a cancer is cut is wholly different from that when fibrous goiters are severed.

These cancers may be distinguished by the border-line between the malignancy and the unaffected gland (Fig. 228). The malignant part extends diffusely into the unaffected part nowhere limited by a capsule. On the other hand, an entire lobe may be involved whereas the opposite lobe is goitrous. One infers in such cases that the malignant lobe was goitrous before the beginning of the malignancy (Fig. 229).

When the malignancy begins within the nodulations of a large goiter it may attain considerable dimensions before it causes any disturbance (Fig. 230). The nodulations of the goiter obstruct palpation of the lesion

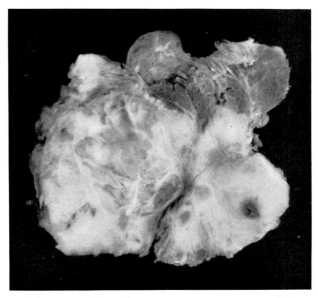

Fig. 228. Carcinoma developing in a thyroid gland not previously goitrous. The lower part is a simple carcinoma while the upper part is a normal gland.

and protect the surrounding structures, notably the trachea, from early invasion by the new growth.

Conversely the invasion may early spread extensively so that the adjacent structures are involved. Most commonly the trachea is earliest invaded, even to a degree causing the formation of a malignant nodule within it, and the esophagus may be so extensively invaded that deglutition becomes impossible and the patient starves to death. The large nerves and vessels of the neck are sometimes invaded (Fig. 231), requiring their removal. Operations of this magnitude are not operations for surgeons, they are technical stunts for beginners. Usually when such specimens are examined in the laboratory it is found that the carotid vessel was not invaded and could have been separated from the vessel.

Histology. Carcinomas having their origin in goiters or a normal gland at first present the appearance of an adenocarcinoma (Fig. 232). The structure may have the structure of a simple cancer or show a diffuse spindleform arrangement.

Squamous cell carcinomas have been described, yet without much justification because one finds transitions to more typically acinal cells. At most one finds masses of large cells, but they lack the typical columnar or nest arrangement of squamous celled cancer (*A*, Fig. 233). The cells

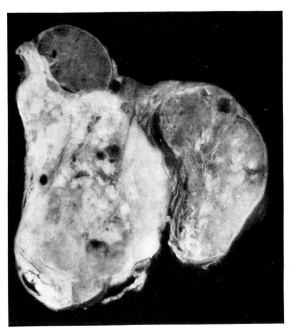

FIG. 229. Diffuse carcinoma involving the entire right lobe save a nodule at the top. The left lobe presented a diffuse colloid goiter.

are large granular nuclei but the protoplasm is ill defined (*B*, Fig. 233). The protoplasm is faintly acidophilic, having this characteristic in common with many forms of cells in a variety of goiters. This type of cell is most generally found in very hard, slowly growing cancers.

MIXED TUMORS

These tumors are corollaries to the malignancies which develop on fetal adenomas. They are microscopically malignant but the surgeon has learned that there probably will be no recurrence after operation. I have chosen this title because of their resemblance, both clinically and pathologically, to the common tumors of the parotid gland.

It is obvious that the group is somewhat ill defined. Its members are worthy of special study because they emphasize their resemblance to

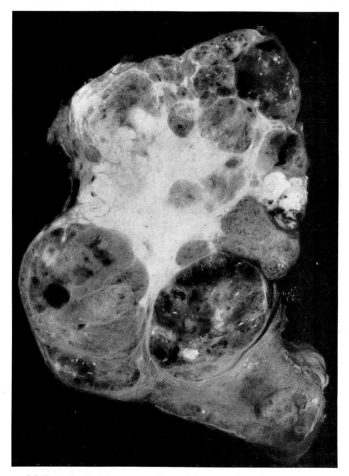

FIG. 230. Malignancy in the center of a nodular goiter.

certain mixed tumors, and the surgeon should know as definitely as possible what he has cured. An understanding of these tumors will make one more alert in removing fetal adenomas as a prophylactic measure. Their study is unequivocally a combined clinical and a laboratory one. Either alone leads only to confusion.

Pathogenesis. Of course these tumors always develop in fetal adenomas. The cellular proliferation is slow and the physical changes are so inconspicuous that the cellular changes may not be suspected until found in the laboratory. The capsule remains intact for long periods. Ultimately no doubt they may become definitely malignant when the capsule is pierced. From then on they develop like the carcinomas previously described.

Pathology. The cross-section presents a surface differing little from that of the fetal adenomas but those in which there is more active pro-

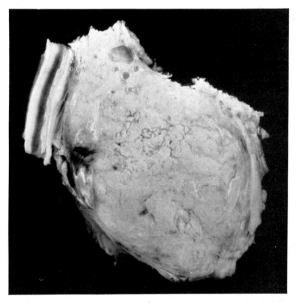

FIG. 231. Carcinoma of the thyroid which had invaded the large nerves and vessels of the neck. The common carotid artery lies at the left of the tumor.

liferation may be whitish, like the definitely malignant, in certain regions. The capsule is everywhere smooth and intact.

Histology. These tumors differ from the more malignant ones in the uniformity of the cells and the tendency to retain a columnar, spherical or papillary arrangement. The more columnar the arrangement of the cells the nearer is the approach to malignancy.

The simplest form presents a papillary tumor extending into the lumen of a cyst (*A*, Fig. 234). A more advanced stage presents solid columns of cells (*B*, Fig. 234). Instead of interlacing columns there may be small acini for the most part without lumina. Each acinus is

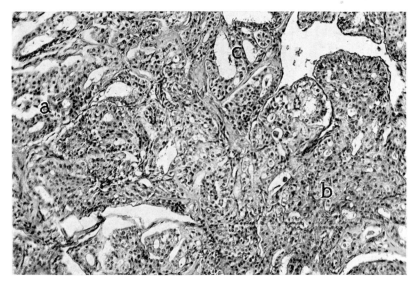

FIG. 232. Early carcinoma of the thyroid gland: *a*, acini preserved, containing lumina but the colloid, if any, is stainless; *b*, solid masses of cells which have lost their uniformity in size and staining; *c*, fairly normal acini containing all but stainless colloid.

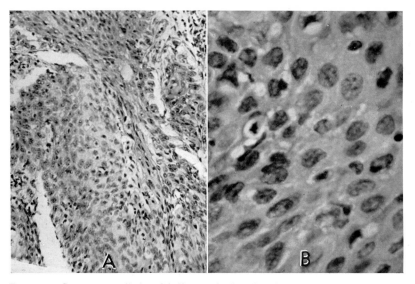

FIG. 233. Squamous celled epithelioma of the thyroid gland: *A*, closely packed large cells more or less diffusely arranged; *B*, the nuclei are large and granular, the protoplasm abundant but more or less suffused with neighboring cells so that in the more degenerated syncytial masses are produced.

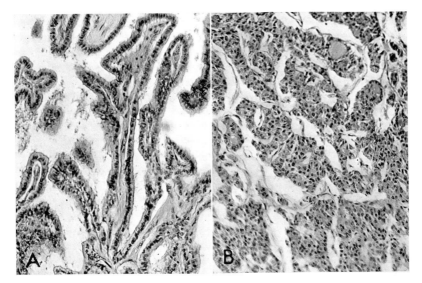

Fig. 234. Mixed tumors of the thyroid gland. *A*, Papillary tumors ending in blunt extremities. *B*, Columns of cells arranged in an interlacing network. The cells remain equal in size and stainability. A few indefinite acini, one with colloid, are visible.

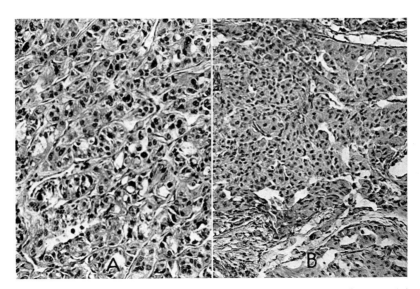

Fig. 235. Mixed tumor of the thyroid gland. *A*, Small acini, very few containing lumina and none colloid. The cells are uniform in size. *B*, More advanced stage in which all semblance to acini is lost and the cells are irregular in size and stainability. A number of vessels are visible. Well 8 years.

surrounded by a distinct layer of fibrous tissue (*A*, Fig. 235). A more advanced stage is represented by the loss of the round arrangement, the cells becoming variable in shape and size (*B*, Fig. 235). Some specimens have a very distinct spindle form. These shake one's confidence in the theory of the connective tissue origin of some of the apparently spindle celled sarcomas.

SARCOMA

There has been much controversy over sarcomas of the thyroid gland. Some eminent pathologists deny that there is any such thing. Be this as

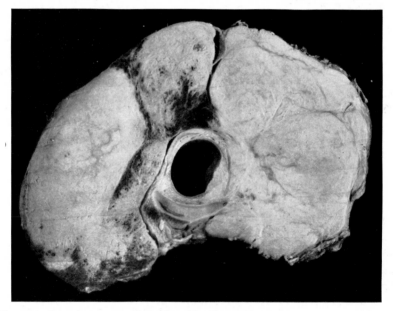

FIG. 236. Lymphosarcoma of the thyroid. The nodular tumor surrounds the trachea and esophagus without compressing either.

it may, one encounteres tumors that run the clinical course of sarcoma, and to the naïve surgeon they look like sarcoma in the laboratory. The surgeon fares better when he slips up on the finer points of pathology than when he blindly accepts the more skilled pathologists' verdicts. In fact too much time has been expended in trying to align certain tumors into the general scheme of things. For instance, in cases of the tumors of the parotid gland there is much controversy regarding what they develop from. The surgeon knows how they act clinically and how they look microscopically. Who cares where they come from—where the patient is going, and when, is the chief concern of the surgeon.

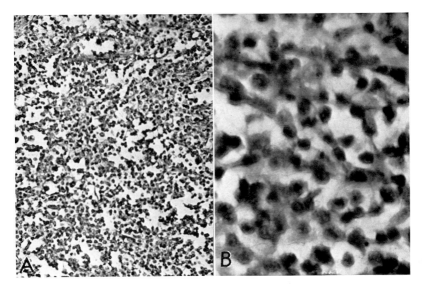

FIG. 237. Lymphosarcoma of the thyroid gland. *A*, Low power shows diffuse arrangement of lymphocytes. *B*, High power: the reticulum surrounds the individual cells. The walls of many of the blood vessels are made up of tumor cells. A few large cells with stainless protoplasm are visible in the lower part.

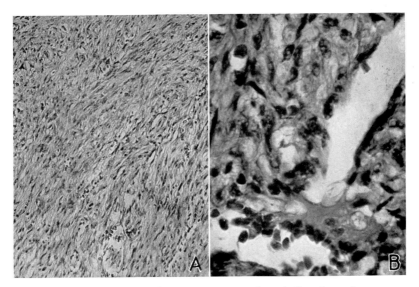

FIG. 238. Fibrosarcoma of the thyroid gland. *A*, The spindle cells are in many areas arranged in whorls. *B*, The more cellular areas show cells of varying sizes and shapes. These cells are in close relation to the walls of the blood vessels.

Therefore certain types of sarcomas will be discussed from the point of view of the surgeon. The first criterion is a pseudo expansile growth of spindle or round cells with intercellular stroma, and metastasis by way of the blood stream.

Pathogenesis. Of the beginnings of sarcoma nothing is known. One finds an enlarged thyroid occupying one or both lobes. Lacking in toxicity and being more or less uniform, Riedel's or Hashimoto's struma is thought of. As it continues to grow, malignancy is suspected; since it is smooth or slightly lobulated and elastic and entirely lacks the density of carcinoma, the diagnosis of sarcoma is the only alternative. The local disturbance of respiration is less pronounced than in carcinomas which are like sarcomas of the gut and preserve the lumina by their expansile growth (Fig. 236). The patient is rapidly reduced and at autopsy metastases, chiefly in the solid organs, are found.

Pathology. In the absence of obstructing signs and due to the extent of the tumor there is usually little urge to attack them surgically and all the pathology is obtained at autopsy.

In less widely involved cases in which the tumor is confined to one lobe, operation is feasible, generally under the diagnosis of a reactive enlargement, above mentioned. Only the smoothness of the tumor and its elasticity make a diagnosis of sarcoma seem plausible. Some of these refuse a definite classification even after laboratory study.

The cross-section shows a surface that is pinkish, sometimes pinkish white. Spheroidal areas are usually seen here and there, with larger lobules making up the mass of the tumor (Fig. 236). Much the same picture may be obtained in the less extensive growths. They are more likely to be whiter in color, and the probable status awaits the histologic examination; then often enough it is not conclusive.

Histology. The most distinctive of these tumors are the lymphosarcomas. The lymphoid-like cells surrounded by a definite stroma and the close relation to the blood vessels make a fairly conclusive picture (Fig. 237). It is impossible to believe these are of epithelial origin. Of course one must think of Hodgkin's disease and diffuse reactive processes. The more fibrous tumors show spindle cells arranged in whorls with more cellular areas interposed (Fig. 238).

Literature

Tumors of the Thyroid Gland. Until the position of fetal adenomas in the tumors of the thyroid gland is more clearly comprehended a discussion of the literature of the genesis of thyroid cancer is more likely to be confusing than clarifying.

In general many excellent papers are available; among these may be mentioned the following: Arons (*Ann. Surg.*, Jan. 1930, 91, 44–56), Curtis and Delaney (*Arch. Path.*,

Oct. 1930 10, 580–586), Clute and Warren (*Am. J. Cancer* Oct. 1931, 15, 2563), D'Abreu (*Brit. J. Surg.*, April 1933, 20, 666) Dunhill (*Ibid.*, July 1931, 19, 83–113), Lahey (*S. Clin. N. Am.*, June 1932, 12, 795–803), Lerman (*M. Clin. N. Am.*, Jan. 1933, 16, 1003), Levi and Hankins (*Am. J. Cancer*, Feb. 1935, 23, 328), Mason and Warren (*Am. J. Path.*, July 1931, 7, 415–422), Pusch and Nelson (*Am. J. Cancer*, April 1935, 23, 791–796), Rice (*ibid.*, July 1931, 15, 2301), Rienhoff and Lewis (*Arch. Surg.*, Jan. 1928, 16, 79–116), Rosenthal and Willis (*J. Coll. Surg. Australasia*, Nov. 1930, 3, 257), Shapiro (*Ann. Surg.*, Dec. 1930, 92, 1031), Smith (*Arch. Path.*, Oct. 1930, 10, 524–530), Smith, Pool and Olcott (*Am. J. Cancer*, Jan. 1934, 20, 1–32), Tinker (*Arch. Surg.*, April 1933, 26, 705–711), Ward and Carr (*Tr. Am. Asso. for Study of Goiter.* July 1930 122–5), Warren (*Arch. Path.*, Feb. 1931, 11, 255–257), Willis (*Am. J. Path.*, May 1931, 7, 187–208) and Wilson (*Ann. Sug.*, August 1921, 74, 129–184).

INDEX